UNDER ATTACK

How an Autoimmune Condition
May Be Sabotaging Your Health
and What You Can Do About It

I0029722

UNDER ATTACK

How an Autoimmune Condition
May Be Sabotaging Your Health
and What You Can Do About It

by Aubry Tager, DNM, DC, BCIM, DAAIM,
ND(anpq)

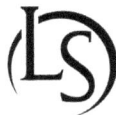

LEON SMITH
PUBLISHING

www.LeonSmithPublishing.com

ISBN: 978-1-945446-17-7

Dedication

To my family.

Acknowledgments

Without certain people, this book and the experiences that led to its creation would not have been possible. I'd like to acknowledge some of those people.

First and foremost, I want to thank my wife, Doree Levine. No one in the world stands behind me and supports me the way that she does.

My children, Zach, Jordyn, and Cooper Tager, are always there to bring a smile to my face and make me an extremely proud father.

I have a relatively small family, including Dr. Sheldon and Rosalie Tager, Carol and Allan Levine, Danny and Jennifer Rosenoff, and Mandy and Adam Rosenoff, and I want to thank them for making me who I am today.

I'd also like to thank my extended family, the Boidmans, Rosenoffs, and Yaphes, and all those who have had faith in me or influenced me greatly in my career.

I want to thank my friend, mentor, and colleague, Dr. Michael Johnson, for making me the doctor that I am today, and Dr. Andy Barlow for being a true teacher, guide, and friend.

My thanks go to Dr. Ted Carrick for getting the ball rolling and then hitting it out of the park with his brilliant teaching on functional neurology, and to Dr. Michael Hall for giving me my first introduction to the world of functional neurology.

My continued interest in functional medicine and functional neurology is being greatly enhanced by the teachings of Dr. Brandon Brock and Dr. Datis Kharrazian.

To Dr. Michael Dorfman and the late Dr. Richard Lutz, I extend a special thank you for launching my career.

I want to thank my many colleagues and friends for their contributions, including Dr. Akiba Green, Dr. Santo Fera, Dr. Alex Liberman, Dr. Ed Beyer, Dr. Thomas Santucci, Dr. Robert Melillo, Drs. Robert Birch and Paola Porrone, Dr. Karl Oliger, Dr.Josh Huffman, Dr. Walter Crooks, Dr. Joel Rosen, Dr. Michael Glickart, and Dr. Rob McCarthy.

My thanks also go to my close friends, Neil Brown, Elanna Peril, Costa Danassis, Matthew Ray, Sandrine Lavalle, and Paige Brodkin. (How could I write a book without mentioning you?)

And finally, I'd like to extend a special thank you to my publishers, editors, and friends, Keith and Maura Leon, for making this project possible.

Table of Contents

Introduction

A CLEAR CHOICE

Why have you decided to pick up this book?

Come on, there must be a reason.

Do you or someone you love suffer from an autoimmune disorder?

Do you have to deal with the daily rigors of these frustrating diseases?

Well, let me tell you, you are not alone.

In the United States, the National Institute of Health estimates up to 23.5 million U.S. citizens suffer from autoimmune (AI) diseases and disorders.

And that number is rising.

> *Researchers have identified 80–100 different diseases and suspect at least forty additional that may have an autoimmune basis. These diseases are chronic and can be life-threatening.*

~ American Autoimmune and Related Diseases Association

So why, then, as a physician and author, did I choose to write about these conditions?

To answer that, let me tell you a little bit about myself.

I was born and raised in Montreal, Canada. At the age of nineteen, I attended the University of Toronto with the intention of becoming a lawyer. Even though I had always been very interested in the body, medicine, and healthcare, I chose to focus on law.

But that changed quickly when I was at university because I was extremely focused on health, nutrition, and exercise. I was a member of the varsity football team. I spent a couple of summers working as an orderly at the Jewish General Hospital in Montreal, during which I became exposed to various areas of healthcare. I worked in the emergency room, orthopedics, and geriatrics. I even worked in areas like psychiatry, where I had to restrain patients who were locked in a secured wing of the hospital.

From my work in that hospital, I realized that I really didn't want to be a lawyer; I wanted to be a doctor.

But what kind of doctor would I be?

I've always been focused on complex things. I'm a problem solver who likes to tackle large challenges. Sometimes, people tell me that I'm focusing on too large of a task. So at first, I thought that if I were going to be a doctor, I would probably be a surgeon.

The problem was that I was also very athletic and passionate about sports. I grew up enjoying activities like skiing, snowmobiling, waterskiing, hockey, tennis, and cycling. I really did not want to give those things up, but I thought I would probably have to if I were going to become a surgeon.

With that in mind, what other options were available?

Based on my background and interests, the options that made the most sense for me were dentistry, podiatry, and chiropractic. I had grown up with a father who was a dentist, and this provided a very nice lifestyle. From his perspective, dentistry offered freedom to spend weekends with family and to travel. But I wasn't overly intrigued by the family dental practice. So that narrowed my choices down to podiatry and chiropractic.

When I asked myself whether I wanted to deal with the feet or the nervous system, the answer was clear. I chose the nervous system.

In 1994, I headed to Parker College of Chiropractic in Dallas, Texas, and that is where my journey began. During my first year of school, I was introduced to Dr. Michael Hall, a chiropractic neurologist. While at that time I did not understand what a chiropractic neurologist was, I was intrigued by his compassion, dedication, and expertise in the field of neurology. I began my studies with Dr. Hall, and he also became my chiropractor.

Through Dr. Hall, I was introduced to Dr. Ted Carrick, who is probably the world's foremost authority on chiropractic neurology. In the limelight over the last couple of years, Dr. Carrick has appeared on television shows such as *Nightline* for treating complex neurologic cases—not typical chiropractic cases but severe neurologic problems. He's the doctor who was recently credited with getting hockey's Sidney Crosby back on the ice, and he has treated many other professional hockey players, including Claude Giroux and Jonathan Toews.

I was fascinated by Dr. Carrick's work, and in 1997, while still a student at Parker, I enrolled in a three-year post-graduate program in chiropractic neurology. The program opened my eyes to new treatment strategies for a multitude of neurologic problems, including closed head injuries and strokes. At that point, we had new tools to offer patients.

After graduating in 1999, I joined the practice of Drs. Richard Lutz and Michael Dorfman in Detroit, Michigan, where I stayed for about six years before moving with my family to Vermont and starting my own practice.

But after a few years in Vermont, it became increasingly difficult to be away from my family of origin. So as the journey to write this book began, I decided to make some geographical changes and relocate to Montreal, Quebec, where the next chapter of life-changing care begins.

My training is as a Doctor of Chiropractic (DC). In addition, I am a Doctor of Natural Medicine (DNM), and I am Board Certified in Integrative Medicine. I also sit on the Executive Committee for the American Association of Integrative Medicine.

Over the past couple of years, I have teamed up with Dr. Michael Johnson, who was in Ted Carrick's program with me at Parker College, although we didn't know each other at the time. Dr. Johnson has integrated all of Dr. Carrick's information, along with the work of a few other doctors, to combine metabolic and neurologic care. Using neuro-metabolic care, we've started to see some profound changes in people's lives. This group of doctors, currently over five hundred strong, is called the Johnson Neuro-Metabolic Super Group.

To find a neuro-metabolic doctor near you, please visit www. LifeChangingCare.com

We focus on autoimmune conditions and other relative neuro-metabolic conditions such as concussion and vertigo. We treat both children and adults with ADHD, autism, and cognitive processing disorders. There is a large overlap in all of these conditions, because they all change the brain's ability to function and affect the body's metabolic processing.

We want to stabilize your autonomic nervous system, balance your brain hemispheres, prevent neurologic degeneration and future changes, stabilize the corrections, and maintain them once they are achieved.

We get referrals from medical doctors, osteopaths, chiropractors, naturopaths, physical therapists, and psychologists, as well as from advertisements, people who are researching things on the Internet, and people who are reading books, like this one. That's how our practice is set up.

My office has a vision, a mission, and a specific set of goals.

- **Our vision** is to be a primary healthcare center, dedicated to optimizing the health and well-being of our patients.

- **Our mission** is to add value to the lives of our patients.

- **Our goals** are to test and treat each patient neurologically, metabolically, and structurally in order to return them to the most optimal state of health possible.

This philosophy was brought to the forefront by Dr. Michael Johnson and Dr. Andy Barlow in Tupelo, Mississippi.

When patients come into my office, these are the things we strive to accomplish.

THE FUNCTIONAL APPROACH

Typical conventional medicine takes a symptom-based approach. There is a remedy for each symptom that you come in with, and that remedy is usually medication. The *Physician's Desk Reference* (PDR) contains all of the medications available in the United States and is updated every year. Canada has an equivalent book, the *Compendium of Pharmaceuticals and Specialties* (CPS). Physicians generally look at your symptoms and then look up those symptoms in the PDR or the Merck manual of differential diagnosis to find the recommended medication.

Some physicians may suggest a medication on a trial basis, even if symptoms don't exactly match those that the medication is meant to treat.

Usually, this is not the best approach for chronic conditions. Medications can have a lot of unpleasant side effects, and since they are filtered out by the liver, repeated use can have ill effects on the liver. It doesn't take long for the damage to occur.

What if you decided to avoid the dangers of medications by seeking alternative care from a practitioner with a different point of view, such as a chiropractor, naturopath, or osteopath?

Most likely, you would still be getting a recommendation for something to treat your symptoms.

For example:

- If you had problems with your mood, an alternative practitioner might recommend that you try some kava kava.

- If you had type 2 diabetes, chromium picolinate might be suggested.

Even though you're getting a natural substance instead of a medication, this is still a symptom-based approach.

With *neuro-metabolic care*, we use a systemic approach, also referred to as *integrative medicine*, *functional medicine*, or *functional neurology*. We look at how the systems of the body are functioning. In the systemic approach, we ask ourselves:

What is causing all of these symptoms, and how can we correct them?

If you're having problems with weight loss, could it be your thyroid?

If it's your thyroid, do we give you thyroid medication?

What are the alternatives?

Should we give you an herb for your thyroid?

Maybe there's a problem with your adrenal glands, liver, or gallbladder. That's a functional, systemic approach—looking at the whole, the larger picture. That's how we approach our patient care, and it's the primary way that integrative medicine differs from conventional medicine or general alternative therapies.

THE IMMUNE SYSTEM, STRESS, AND INFLAMMATION

At the age of fifteen, I was diagnosed with type 1 diabetes and had to change my life instantly. I did not have a choice; if I didn't change, I would die.

At the time (the mid-1980s), alternative treatments and nutrition were not what they are today. Information was not available, technology was different, and there were no specialized diets or even diet options for things like soft drinks and desserts.

As challenging as this was for me as a teenager, I embraced the lifestyle of exercise and nutrition and moved forward without any major difficulties. Because of this experience, I developed an interest in healthcare, which ultimately led to my specific interest in autoimmune conditions.

What is an autoimmune condition?

When your immune system mistakes something in your body for a foreign invader, it attacks your own body. It will attack any tissues in your body, not just one specific tissue. It may attack enzymes, the nervous system, or in the case of diabetes, it can attack what's called the *islets of Langerhans*, which are the cells in the pancreas that produce insulin.

Autoimmune conditions can affect your:

- Thyroid
- Blood

- Gastrointestinal tract
- Nerves
- Lungs
- Skin
- Muscles
- Bones
- Brain

An autoimmune condition doesn't just attack one area of your body, like your pancreas or your thyroid; it can attack multiple areas. It can, essentially, attack your entire body.

It can:

- Attack your pancreas, causing diabetes

- Attack your gut or your stomach lining, causing irritable bowel syndrome (IBS) or Crohn's disease

- Attack your joints, causing ailments like rheumatoid arthritis or psoriatic arthritis

- Attack your brain and spinal cord, causing multiple sclerosis

In this book, we're going to look at what happens to different parts of the body with each one of these conditions.

What triggers autoimmune conditions?

They can be triggered by:

- Stress
- Hormones
- Heavy metals
- Food
- Pesticides and poisons

When your body's own natural immune system—which normally fights off problems coming into your body—attacks a part of itself instead, that's an immune system problem. Therefore, it's your immune system that needs to be healed.

Stress that sends your immune system out of balance can be:

- Physical
- Chemical
- Emotional

Physical stress could result from:

- A car accident
- A trauma
- A fall
- A sports-related injury
- Any other physical injury

Chemical stress can be a reaction to:

- A specific medication
- A chemical that you've been exposed to

Emotional stress could be caused by:

- The loss of a loved one
- The loss of a job
- The loss of money

These are all stressors on the body. When your immune system goes out of balance because of these stressors, this imbalance can become dominant and attack your own body.

There are specific tests we can run to see if your immune system is out of balance. If you have an autoimmune condition, you need to be tested to see what's causing it to happen.

One of the main things we see with any autoimmune condition is an active *antigen*.

An antigen could be:

- A parasite
- A virus or a bacteria
- A mold
- Certain foods

Once an antigen is introduced into the body, one of the major changes that can be seen in the neuro-metabolic system is inflammation. Inflammation is a huge factor when dealing with autoimmune conditions.

What is inflammation?

Generally speaking, *inflammation* is the vascular tissue (blood vessels) responding to injury. *Acute inflammation* means that it's happening immediately in response to an injury.

An acute injury could be:

- Hitting your finger with a hammer
- Stubbing your toe
- Falling when you're skiing

In response to an injury, blood flows to the surface, and you experience the cardinal signs of inflammation.

The cardinal signs are:

- Pain
- Redness
- Swelling
- Heat
- Loss of function

This is an acute inflammatory response to anything that injures the tissues. It can happen to your central nervous system, your skin, or any organ in your body.

Why?

It's a defense mechanism for injury. The increased blood flow gives you more plasma protein to remove the cause of the problem.

If this becomes a chronic condition, you'll end up having inflammation throughout your body. That doesn't mean you're going to be walking around all hot and red, looking like a balloon, but the tissues inside your body are going to be inflamed, and inflammation makes it harder to get better.

How do we treat the inflammation?

Your Gut and Your Nervous System

In treating inflammation, one of the main areas we'll focus on is the gut.

What, exactly, is your gut?

Your gut is made up of several components, for example:

- Stomach
- Duodenum
- Small intestine
- Large intestine

It is estimated that 80 percent of your immune system is in your gut. Your gut contains trillions of bacteria, and in order for your body to heal properly, we have to make sure that the good bacteria outnumber the bad ones.

But what does this bacteria have to do with neurology?

Is there a correlation between your brain and your gut?

Yes, there is.

The muscles that push food along your gastrointestinal tract, like all of the muscles in your body, contain electrical activity — called *action potentials*—which cause the contraction of the muscles. When one of these muscles is stimulated, every one of the muscles in that network will be stimulated. The muscles in your stomach and gastrointestinal tract are influenced by your autonomic nervous system.

Your autonomic nervous system has two branches:

1. Sympathetic
2. Parasympathetic

Your sympathetic nervous system is responsible for your fight-or-flight response. It's concerned with getting you out of the way of something dangerous.

If you see a tiger coming toward you or a police car chasing you with the siren on, what happens to your body?

Your blood pressure rises, your pupils dilate, and you're in fight-or-flight mode. This is an automatic response, brought on by a reaction from your sympathetic nervous system.

Your parasympathetic nervous system is responsible for your rest-and-digest response.

Can you run down the street and eat a sandwich at the same time?

No, you can't.

You have to be able to rest and digest. When you do this, you are using your parasympathetic nervous system.

The movement of food in your gastrointestinal tract is called *intestinal motility*, or *peristalsis*. Messages from your brain stimulate different parts of your nervous system to send messages down to your gut. If there are problems in your nervous system, your gut won't function properly. When your gut doesn't function properly, then you can develop problems with your immune system.

At the junction of your esophagus and the top of your stomach, there is a muscle called the *lower esophageal sphincter*, which prevents your stomach acid from coming back up into your esophagus. In order for that to work, you need to have a stomach pH in the range of two to three. If the pH is not low enough—because you don't have enough acid in your stomach—then your lower esophageal sphincter will stay open and allow acid to come back up. New research suggests that generally, this would be in the form of lactic acid and would be experienced as *heartburn*.

If you don't have enough stomach acid to break down the food in your stomach, it's called *hypochlorhydria*. *Hypo* means less than, and *chlorhydria* is stomach acid, so *hypochlorhydria* occurs when you have less than the optimal amount of stomach acid. When this occurs, as is very common with autoimmune conditions such as Hashimoto's and diabetes, there is a lack of stomach acid in the stomach, or if you prefer, a decrease in gasrtic acid secretion.

If you ask the average person what causes heartburn they'll likely tell you it's from too much acid. That is the impression that most of us are left with after watching commercials selling antacids or visits to doctors within the HMO/PPO system who prescribe H2 antagonists and proton pump inhibitors. These are much stronger drugs that severely diminish your body's process of making hydrochloric acid.

Because the stomach has to contain the very strong acid HCL, it requires a barrier so the cells of the stomach don't get digested immediately and ulcerate. Within the stomach, the body creates a protective barrier, mostly through mucous and bicarbonate.

The whole key to understanding how *low* stomach acid could possibly cause heartburn, GERD, or acid reflux, is in understanding what current research tells us about the one-way valve referred to as the *Lower Esophageal Sphincter*, or LES.

When a person has low stomach acid and the pH doesn't reach the level of acidity to trigger the closing of the LES, the LES stays open. At that point, whatever acid is in the stomach, even if not very strong, that comes in contact with the esophagus can cause damage and what you know as heartburn, reflux, or GERD ensues.

This mechanism accounts for approximately 80 percent of heartburn, reflux, and GERD.

Other conditions that inhibit the LES from closing normally include:

- Obesity
- Bacterial overgrowth
- Diaphragmatic dysfunction
- Pregnancy

Antacids further inhibit the body's natural ability to produce necessary levels of hydrochloric acid. Having strong stomach acid levels gives us the best chance to stay healthy and free from infections like H. Pylori, E. Coli, Hepatitis A, or common parasites like roundworm, which are not uncommon for us to see in patients with metabolic disorders.

Infections from bacteria, viruses or parasites within the digestive tract can also be triggers or drivers in autoimmune conditions. They can also cause systemic inflammation and can often be difficult to identify.

HCL is fundamentally required for the absorption of minerals and vitamins like:

- Calcium
- Magnesium
- Zinc
- Iron
- Copper
- Vitamin C
- Vitamin K
- Vitamin B

Bacterial infections have been implicated in conditions like:

- Allergic reactions
- Autoimmune and other inflammatory diseases

By causing an impairment of the intestinal barrier, infections compromise the tight little junctions that normally keep food from leaking out. Once food leaks out, you have *leaky gut syndrome*, which causes a problem not just in your gut, but also throughout your entire body. For more about leaky gut syndrome, see the chapter on gastroinestinal disorders.

Some of the main causes of leaky gut are reactions to these foods:

- Gluten
- Dairy

- Soy
- Corn

These are the main causes of inflammatory responses in the body. Generally, once gluten and other inflammatory foods are removed from the diet, the intestine can resume its normal barrier function, autoantibodies are normalized, and the autoimmune process shuts off.

This demonstrates how one specific little circumstance — in this case, making sure that you have enough stomach acid and a functioning gut — can help you prevent or heal an autoimmune condition.

A study performed by University of Alberta's Dr. Bruce Yacyshyn and colleagues demonstrated that 25 percent of multiple sclerosis patients have increased intestinal permeability (Yacyshyn et al., 1994). It also showed that both patients with MS and patients with Crohn's disease have an increased number of peripheral B cells (lymphocytes that make antibodies), indicating that people who have a genetic predisposition and have these cells in their stomachs are more at risk of MS and Crohn's disease.

Autoimmune diseases have a multifactorial nature. Their antecedents (precursors) can include:

- Genetics
- Dietary factors
- Environmental factors
- Occupational factors
- Learned behavior
- Traumatic factors
- Disease-induced factors
- Drug-induced factors

There is no one major cause for all autoimmune conditions, and you can be born predisposed to a specific condition, but that doesn't mean that it's going to happen. The triggering factors can be genetic, environmental, or both.

Possible triggers include:

- Trauma
- Microbes
- Antigens
- Toxins
- Radiation
- Drugs
- Immune response

To support nutritional balance and decrease the inflammation, we look at your gastrointestinal function, structure, and energy production, and we evaluate you with the following questions:

Do you have any kind of oxidative stress going on?

How is your mind-body connection?

How is your neuroendocrine system functioning?

Your Adrenals and Thyroid

Your adrenal glands are located above your kidneys, and there's one on each side. These are the glands that respond to stress.

There are two parts to your adrenal glands:

- The adrenal cortex
- The adrenal medulla

The *adrenal cortex* is a layer of tissue around the outside of the adrenals. It produces glucocorticoids and mineralocorticoids, which we call aldosterone, and androgens — primarily dehydroepiandrosterone (DHEA) and androstenedione.

The physiological relationship between your brain's hypothalamus, your pituitary, and your adrenals is extremely important because they all communicate with one another. The communication loop goes through your upper and mid-brainstem, down into your gut, and back up again to your brain. All of these areas, working in concert, must function properly.

The *adrenal medulla* is the interior of the adrenal glands. It's important mainly in releasing epinephrine, norepinephrine, and cortisol, the major products released in response to the fight-or-flight sympathetic reaction. If the adrenal glands release too much cortisol in response to stressful situations, then cortisol becomes toxic to your brain.

If they're not functioning properly, the adrenal glands can cause secondary problems, such as Addison's disease, another autoimmune condition. Secondary diseases can result from a lack of stimulation by the pituitary or the hypothalamus. If your adrenal glands aren't regulated, there's a greater potential for problems in other areas.

Your thyroid gland is known as *the Master Gland* of the body. Your thyroid has two lobes and is located in the front part of your neck, just below your Adam's apple.

Your thyroid produces two main hormones:

- Thyroxine (T4)
- Triiodothyronine (T3)

The T_4 hormone is required for normal brain development and function, and T_3 is the usable form. Most of the conversion from T_4 to T_3 (60 to 70 percent) occurs in the liver. If you're having symptoms that look like a thyroid problem, it may not be solely your thyroid. There might be problems with your liver, gallbladder, or other parts of your endocrine system. But it's extremely important to consider your thyroid as well.

Oxidation

When someone mentions your body's pH, to what are they referring?

There are several places in your body where pH can be measured. The pH of your stomach, for example, is a bit different from the pH of your body's extracellular fluid (ECF), and the pH of your blood is completely different from the first two. If your medical doctor tells you that pH doesn't matter or doesn't change, then they're probably referring to blood pH. What we're concerned with here is the pH of your extracellular fluid, not your blood. The optimum range for that pH is between 6.4 and 7.0.

To measure pH, we look for the normal hydrogen ion concentration. Since every cell in your body already produces acid, eating foods that are more acidic can cause problems. You are constantly vulnerable to changes in your pH. If it fluctuates, you're going to be susceptible to numerous systemic problems, so it's important to make sure that your pH is in check. There are many protocols we can use to help stabilize your pH level.

While the very process of living and breathing produces oxygen stress, environmental stressors and toxicity increase the demands on your body's antioxidant mechanism. We need to encourage antioxidation and anti-inflammatory functions in your body to minimize those global effects. Long-term inflammation and pro-oxidant activity that is not balanced by antioxidants can lead to other problems, such as atherosclerosis (ASVD), liver problems, and diabetes.

Most detoxification occurs in the liver. If the pathways are not functioning properly and your liver is not able to detoxify everything, then you'll end up having long-term problems.

The most powerful antioxidant in your body is glutathione. It neutralizes free radicals, detoxifies your liver, and supports your immune system, nervous system, gastrointestinal system, and lungs. While glutathione is normally present in your body, there are times when it can be depressed. We can run specific tests to determine whether enough glutathione is being processed in your body.

Making Informed Choices

In this book, we'll look at specific autoimmune conditions, how they affect specific areas of your body, and what kinds of approaches you can take that might be different from what you are doing right now.

I try not to put labels on my patients. When I treat you, I'm treating a person, not a disease process. Whatever conditions you present with, those are what I'm going to treat. I'm not treating you because you happen to fall into a specific category. The only reason why we're dividing these autoimmune conditions into different categories in this book is because that's how people are relating to it and able to identify with it.

I'm not giving you this information so that you can say, "My doctor doesn't know anything."

And although there is a tremendous amount of medical information here, this is not meant to be a reference book for medical students.

My main purpose is to inform you and give you the opportunity to ask yourself:

As a patient, are there options available to me that I have not been exposed to?

What can I do to change my health for the better with minimal side effects?

I want to make sure that you get the greatest gain without harming your body in the process. I want you to get the right information and leave no stone unturned, so that you can make the best treatment choices for your body.

1

Diabetes

TYPES AND CAUSES

A month before my sixteenth birthday, my parents were out of town, and I was staying with my grandparents. I had not been feeling well for about a week. I thought that I had the flu. Over the course of the week, I had lost over twenty-five pounds. I was feeling quite lethargic.

Throughout the weekend, I hadn't been eating much, but I was incredibly thirsty despite drinking a tremendous amount of liquid. I remember going through at least four or five 2-liter bottles of ginger ale, plus diet cola, orange juice, and whatever else I could get my hands on. I was waking up three or four times in the middle of the night to quench my thirst. I didn't know what was going on.

On Monday morning, back at home, we called the doctor. Not out of any concern — but simply because he was too busy to see me in his office — the doctor told us that it would probably be best if we just went to the hospital.

When we arrived at the hospital, they examined me right away. Within minutes, they determined that my blood sugar level was a whopping 980 milligrams per deciliter (mg/dL), and they told me that I should be dead. They couldn't understand how I had survived. Normal blood sugars at that time were thought to be 80–120 mg/dL.

Within thirty minutes, I was in the intensive care unit. I stayed in the hospital for a week. I found out that I had type 1 diabetes. This meant an instantaneous life change for me. I was told that I had to forget everything I had learned up until that day, beginning with my eating habits. I met with nurse educators who specialized in diabetes. They retrained me in how to eat and started me on insulin therapy.

Back in 1987, the process of determining how much insulin you needed was a guesstimate, and you had to check your blood glucose all the time. We now have more technologically advanced meters for reading the blood glucose levels, but back in the 1980s they were bulky and inaccurate compared to today's technology. Some methods for verifying blood glucose levels used color strips, called *Chemstrips*, which required you to basically just eyeball your reading compared to a color chart.

Initially, I was taking a couple of injections each day, but that didn't work very well. I continued getting educated and tested, including tests for my pancreas to make sure that it was working properly. It turned out that my pancreas was not working at all.

The stress test for the pancreas is called a *glucose tolerance test*. In this procedure, the patient is fed pure glucose drinks and monitored in the hospital for three to four hours in order to see how the pancreas reacts to stress that the glucose drink places on it.

The pancreas is the part of your system that monitors and controls your blood sugar levels. Because my pancreas had not been functioning properly, I have been insulin dependent since 1987. I am currently on an insulin pump to manage my blood sugar levels. I also exercise quite vigorously and frequently, follow a rather strict gluten-free, low-carbohydrate diet, and I take nutritional supplements.

What is Diabetes?

There are two types of diabetes:

1. Diabetes mellitus type 1 (formerly known as *juvenile diabetes* or *child-onset diabetes*)

2. Diabetes type 2 (formerly known as *noninsulin-dependent* or *adult-onset diabetes*)

Diabetes is a resistance to the hormone insulin, which is secreted from a part of your pancreas—tiny cells, called the *islets of Langerhans*. The insulin they secrete helps to normalize your blood sugar level. For your body to function properly, it needs the right amount of glucose, or sugar, in your blood; and for your brain to function properly, you need the right amount of glucose and oxygen. Too much or too little glucose will inhibit proper function. It's all about maintaining equilibrium.

Glucose is used for energy.

There are two kinds:

1. Glucose from the food that you eat
2. Glycogen, which is stored in your liver

For many years people have believed that the only source of fuel for the body, and more specifically the brain, was glucose. We now know that there is another option: *ketones*.

Ketones are a by-product of acetone and beta-hydroxybutyrate. A diet based on this form of fuel was originally developed at the Mayo Clinic for the purposes of treating patients suffering from epilepsy. Over the years it has been shown to be an extremely effective way of losing fat quickly and effectively.

Ketones have also been shown:

- To have a very profound stabilizing effect on blood sugar levels

- To decrease HDL cholesterol

- To decrease triglycerides

- To lower glycosolated hemoglobin

- To lower c-reactive protein, the marker for inflammation leading to heart disease

Diets such as the Atkins diet have been successful in utilizing the principles behind a ketogenic diet. The main principle is an extremely low carbohydrate diet, which allows the body to shift from utilizing carbohydrates as a fuel source and turning to fat instead.

Your body will use other good fats for fuel, such as:

- Coconut oil
- Olive Oil
- Avocados

It will then also burn excess stores of fat in the body as fuel as well, thereby resulting in weight loss.

This type of diet is one of the diets that I recommend to diabetics and others with issues from dysglycemia because it decreases the ebbs and flows of poorly controlled blood sugar levels and the extra release of insulin, which itself is a fat-storing hormone.

How Do You Get Diabetes?

While the question of what causes type 1 diabetes has had many theories but no definitive answer, the research done over the last fifty years seems to point to some form of autoimmune reaction.

How does this autoimmune reaction happen?

It could possibly be a reaction to factors such as antibiotics, immunization, and allergy shots. If your body becomes immune to these things or attacks itself, it could begin to destroy the parts of your pancreas that produce insulin, causing those cells to stop insulin production.

Initially the cells in your body become resistant to insulin. This means that glucose cannot be transported into the cells. This insulin resistance, if continued, could eventually lead to full-blown diabetes. Diabetes will also cause an increase in inflammation and a decrease in the production and release of neurotransmitters such as dopamine, serotonin and gamma amino buteric acid (GABA). Excessive insulin also leads to the formation and storage of fat.

With type 1 diabetes, there is minimal production of insulin or none at all.

With type 2 diabetes, the pancreas is still functioning, but it's not functioning properly. Instead of moving insulin into your cells, it stores the sugar in your blood.

Type 2 diabetes is common in people who eat too much, are overweight or obese, and don't exercise. Too much physical stress on the body, brought on by too much sugar and not controlling what you eat, can bring on type 2 diabetes. It can also be inherited, but it can skip generations. In contrast, type 1 diabetes is not generally hereditary, but the gene for autoimmunity is.

SYMPTOMS, RISKS, AND COMPLICATIONS

Type 2 diabetes is preventable. Even if you have the gene in your family, as long as that gene is not expressed, you won't have to deal with the effects of disease. It's all about managing your eating and exercise.

Symptoms of Diabetes

The two initial symptoms are:

1. Excessive thirst
2. Excessive urination

An excess of sugar in your bloodstream causes fluid to be pulled out of your tissues, making you extremely thirsty to replenish that fluid. As you drink everything in sight, you end up urinating a lot. You start to lose weight through the urine because you're in a state of *ketoacidosis,* and you're spilling ketones.

Ketoacidosis is a condition in which abnormal quantities of ketones are produced in an unregulated biochemical situation. In order to reach a state of ketoacidosis, the body has to be in a state of not producing enough insulin to regulate the flow of fatty acids and the creation of ketone bodies.

Other symptoms of both type 1 and type 2 diabetes include:

- Extreme fatigue
- Irritability
- Blurred vision
- Double vision (or seeing little dots or floaters)
- Confusion
- Dizziness
- Extremely dry mouth (due to all of the liquid being pulled out of your cells)

Risk Factors Associated with Diabetes

What are the risk factors associated with diabetes?

Excess weight: If you are extremely overweight, you could become a type 2 diabetic, especially if you have a family history of diabetes.

Fat Distribution: Being overweight doesn't necessarily mean that you're going to become diabetic. The indicator is where your body is storing the fat. Having a lot of fat around your midsection increases your risk of developing type 2 diabetes.

Inactivity: In North America, there is a preponderance of sedentary living. If you're sitting around watching television and playing video games instead of getting out and exercising, you are increasing your risk of developing type 2 diabetes.

Family History: Even if you don't have a genetic predisposition toward diabetes, your family history can still put you at risk. And if you do have that gene—whether or not it has been expressed—your family history will be a determining factor in your risk of developing type 2 diabetes.

Race: Cultural factors must also be acknowledged and recognized in order to properly address them. Native Americans, Mexican Americans, and some Central Americans, for example, tend to eat a lot of corn, and the corn widely available today—usually genetically modified, unlike the corn their ancestors ate—puts a lot of stress on the pancreas. These cultures are showing a higher predisposition to developing type 2 diabetes. In addition to the stress created by eating corn, eating a lot of fructose, which is derived from corn, will put even more stress on your pancreas.

Complications of Diabetes

You might be thinking:

I'm fine. I don't really have to deal with it.

What's the big deal about not controlling my blood sugar level?

What could possibly happen if I don't control it?

The following are possible complications of diabetes, along with the problems that can be caused by these complications.

Alzheimer's Disease: One of the complications of diabetes is cognitive impairment. The January 2014 issue of the *Journal of Neurology* mentioned a study that showed an increased risk of Alzheimer's disease and cognitive impairment for people who don't have stabilized blood sugar levels (Huang, 2014). If you keep on doing what you've always done and don't take steps to control your blood sugar levels, you could be putting yourself at risk.

Peripheral Neuropathy: A noticeable and prevalent complication is peripheral neuropathy. *Periphery* means away from center, and *neuropathy* is a disease of the nerves.

There are two kinds of neuropathy:

1. *Mononeuropathy*, in which only one nerve is affected
2. *Polyneuropathy*, in which multiple nerves are affected

Diabetes causes polyneuropathy.

People with diabetes are predisposed to having blood vessel problems. The accumulation of glucose in the smaller blood vessels causes those blood vessels and the accompanying nerves to malfunction and can result in abnormal blood pressure.

Other problems associated with peripheral neuropathy can develop.

Amputation: Amputation is common in people who have diabetes. Blood vessel issues can cause problems in the feet and the hands and lead to even bigger problems, like amputation of the toes, foot, or leg.

Since the neuropathy goes *away* from the center, any nerves that go to the small organs—such as your eyes, your bladder, and your sexual organs—can be affected as well. That's one of the reasons why it's so important to control your blood sugar levels.

Erectile Dysfunction: The reason there are so many advertisements for drugs like Viagra® and Cialis® is because diabetes is causing erectile dysfunction in men due to the impairment of the blood vessels of the male genitalia.

Incontinence and Constipation: Peripheral neuropathy can also cause problems with the muscle movement of your internal organs, like your bladder and bowels, which can result in incontinence and constipation.

Blindness: Another big complication with peripheral neuropathy in people who have diabetes is eye problems. I get myself checked by both an ophthalmologist and an optometrist a couple of times a year to make sure that the blood vessels in my eyes are not causing diabetic retinopathy, which could lead to blindness.

Injuries: Peripheral neuropathy from diabetes can cause you to lose your ability to sense temperature and pain, which can put you at risk for injuries. You could put your hand down on a hot glass stovetop and not even realize that it's on because you can't feel anything in your hands or fingers. I've seen many cases like this in which patients got burned.

CONVENTIONAL TREATMENT

How do you take care of diabetes?

What do you do for it?

Blood Sugar Monitoring

If you have Type 1 Diabetes, you're probably going to be taking insulin, so you'll need to understand how to monitor and control your blood sugar level and what type of insulin to take.

How do you monitor your blood sugar level?

You can get a glucose monitor at your local pharmacy. There are different types and brands, and they're fairly inexpensive. Your level should be in the range of 85 to 100 milligrams per deciliter (mg/dL).

Now, because many doctors are going by what's called a pathological range, they'll tell you that a normal blood sugar level is anywhere from 75 to 120 mg/dL.

What would these doctors say if you presented with a blood sugar level of 120?

They'd be likely to tell you, "Your blood sugar level is a little high, but since you're not diabetic, we'll wait to see if you become diabetic, and then, if you do, we can address it with insulin or some other form of medication."

That's crazy!

Why would you wait until you had a problem before you addressed it?

I don't understand why some healthcare providers give this advice.

With a blood sugar level of 120, you'd be experiencing insulin resistance, which would mean that things were not functioning properly. That's why, with a functional medicine approach, we would go for the tighter range.

If your blood sugar level is consistently below 85 or above 100, you're either *hypoglycemic* (your blood sugar is too low) or *hyperglycemic* (your blood sugar level is too high). If you're hyperglycemic, then you're insulin resistant, which means that the insulin is not getting absorbed. You need to address that by monitoring your blood sugar level on a daily basis, so that you don't become diabetic.

Your red blood cells live for 120 days, and their glucose concentration is identified by the measurement of your *glycosylated hemoglobin* (hemoglobin A1C). Throughout the life of your red blood cells, your glycosylated hemoglobin should be between 4.8 and 5.6. If it's higher than that, there's a potential for diabetes, so you should monitor it on a daily basis.

Once insulin resistance or diabetes is discovered, what are the treatment options?

What can you do?

Visit a Specialist: If you or your primary care provider suspects diabetes of any kind, you should first follow up with a doctor (MD or DO) who specializes in the treatment of diabetes. These specialists usually are designated as either Internal Medicine or Endocrinology.

Insulin: For type 1 diabetes, insulin will be prescribed to make up for the insulin that is not being produced by your pancreas. It will come in the form of either an injection or an insulin pump (which automatically pumps insulin into your body throughout the day).

For type 2 diabetes, there are many different kinds of medication, including metformin — sold with the brand names Glucophage, Avandia, and Actos. These medications are believed to increase the effectiveness of the release of insulin from the islets of Langerhans to improve cellular absorption.

THE NATURAL APPROACH

Apart from medication, what else can you do?

The following are my recommendations for naturally supporting your body's ability to heal.

Supplements

Vitamin B Complex: To support your health and to help with any kind of neuropathy, I recommend vitamin B complex. One product that I use myself and recommend for my patients is *Max B-ND* from Premier Research Labs, which has live-source B vitamins for maximum liver, brain, energy, and mood support to aid the nerves and help prevent neuropathy.

Vitamin C: To reduce complications with vision, including diabetic retinopathy, I recommend a minimum of 1,000 milligrams (mg) of vitamin C per day — the most natural source you can find, containing no binders or fillers.

Vitamin D3: People with diabetes are prone to infection because their healing is affected by autoimmunity. If your immune system is not functioning properly, vitamin D3 can help by increasing *cathelicidins*, which fight viruses and bacteria. It can also help with gum disease and other healing problems, such as ulcers.

Because I think that the U.S. government's recommended daily allowance (RDA) of 1,000 international units (IU) isn't enough,

I recommend that all my patients take 5,000 to 10,000 IU of vitamin D3 daily. At 5,000 IU, we start seeing more clinical changes to indicate that it's making in impact. Once again, find a source without binders or fillers.

Vitamin D3 is especially important for people who live in places, like the northern United States and Canada, where they have much less exposure to sunlight during the winter months than people living closer to the equator, in Hawaii, or southern Florida, for example.

Vitamin E: When an autoimmune condition like diabetes occurs, your body produces an excessive amount of free radicals, which can cause cancer and other diseases. Vitamin E is an important antioxidant to decrease the amount of free radicals and inflammation in your body and help you heal faster. It will also help control your blood sugar levels.

Magnesium: Magnesium decreases insulin resistance by allowing insulin to get into your cells more effectively.

Alpha Lipoic Acid: Alpha lipoic acid is an important antioxidant and enzyme co-factor. In cell culture, alpha-lipoic acid — in its reduced form, dihydrolipoic acid — protects neurons against oxidative damage catalyzed by iron or beta amyloid. Beta amyloid proteins are found in people suffering from Alzheimer's disease.

Chromium: Chromium comes in two different forms, *chromium picolinate* and *chromium polynicotinate*. While you may have been told that chromium picolinate is a very effective alternative treatment for controlling blood sugar levels, my research indicates that chromium polynicotinate is much more effective in helping insulin get into your cells.

Nitric Balance: For all of my patients with peripheral neuropathy, I recommend the product *Nitric Balance* from Apex Energetics. It contains *nitric oxide* (not to be confused with *nitrous oxide*), which is extremely beneficial in dilating your capillaries to allow blood to your extremities to flow properly.

Curcumin: Any time you have an autoimmune reaction, it's because there is an increase in inflammatory process throughout your entire body. The more you can decrease the inflammatory response, the more favorable your reaction to treatment will be and the more likely you'll get better. I prefer to use a liposomal curcumin as this form of supplement is the most easily absorbed and effective delivery of curcumin.

Unlike pharmaceutical anti-inflammatories, like ibuprofen, this anti-inflammatory decreases the inflammation in your body globally, without any side effects.

Peripheral Neuropathy Rehab Therapy (PNRT)

Did you know that 80 percent of your brain's function is to inhibit sensory input that could be harmful to your body?

This sensory input is inhibited by your body's large-diameter afferent pathways. When these pathways are not functioning properly due to problems caused by diabetes or injury, your body loses its ability to block out pain, resulting in a loss of your ability to feel subtle vibration and light touch, and you experience numbness, tingling, or pain in your extremities.

To restore this function, I recommend *Peripheral Neuropathy Rehab Therapy* (PNRT). In my office, we use a machine called the *ReBuilder*, which helps to rebuild the axon part of the nerve as well as open the large-diameter afferent pathways to restore the body's ability to inhibit pain.

Laser

Cold laser provides the following benefits:

- Speeds up cell reproduction and decreases the time it takes for healthy new tissue and cells to form and heal.

- Promotes faster healing. The laser stimulates *fibroblasts*, which are needed for damaged tissues to heal. Think of them as the foundation of healing. This will likely speed up the recovery process.

- Increases metabolic activity. Helps the body increase its output of specific enzymes, induces oxygen to blood cells, and helps to create a more effective immune response.

- Reduces the formation of *fibrous tissue*, the type of tissue that could lead to scar formation.

- Reduces inflammatory action. Cold laser reduces swelling caused by inflammation of joints and improves joint mobility. This is very important in relieving pain, especially in the extremities such as the hands, feet, and knees, all problem areas for neuropathy.

- Increases vascular and nerve activity. The laser stimulates lymphatic circulation, which is essential for healing and blood circulation. It allows the affected tissues to have the best possible circulation. It may also help stimulate nerve function.

- Increases the firing of nerves that get damaged by neuropathy.

Dietary Choices

How do you control diabetes with the foods you eat?

Avoiding High-GI Foods: First, it's important to look at the glycemic index (GI) number of the foods that you're choosing. This ranking will give you an indication of the how quickly a particular type of food will be metabolized in your bloodstream relative to other foods. It can help you understand how the sugars and carbohydrates from foods like pasta, corn, and bread are used in your body. The lower the GI number, the more slowly the food will be absorbed in your body, and the higher the GI number, the more quickly it will be absorbed.

If you were to consume something high in sugar, like a soft drink, you would immediately have a spike in your blood sugar level. If your body didn't have the insulin to counteract it, that high blood sugar could lead to complications from hyperglycemia. If this were to continue over an extended period of time, it could even cause you to go into a coma or die.

Choosing foods that have a lower GI ranking will ensure that the sugars in those foods will have a sustained release over a long period of time, and the best foods for that are the ones that are high in fiber.

FOOD	Glycemic index (glucose = 100)	Serving size (grams)	Glycemic load per serving
BAKERY PRODUCTS AND BREADS			
Banana cake, made with sugar	47	60	14
Banana cake, made without sugar	55	60	12
Sponge cake, plain	46	63	17
Vanilla cake made from packet mix with vanilla frosting (Betty Crocker)	42	111	24
Apple cake, made with sugar	44	60	13
Apple cake, made without sugar	48	60	9
Waffles, Aunt Jemima® (Quaker Oats)	76	35	10
Bagel, white, frozen	72	70	25
Baguette, white, plain	95	30	15
Coarse barley bread, 75-80% kernels, average	34	30	7
Hamburger bun	61	30	9
Kaiser roll	73	30	12
Pumpernickel bread	56	30	7
50% cracked wheat kernel bread	58	30	12
White wheat flour bread	71	30	10
Wonder® bread, average	73	30	10
Whole wheat bread, average	71	30	9
100% Whole Grain® bread (Natural Ovens)	51	30	7
Pita bread, white	68	30	10
Corn tortilla	52	50	12
Wheat tortilla	30	50	8
BEVERAGES			
Coca Cola®, average	63	250 mL	16
Fanta®, orange soft drink	68	250 mL	23
Lucozade®, original (sparkling glucose drink)	95 ±10	250 mL	40

Apple juice, unsweetened, average	44	250 mL	30
Cranberry juice cocktail (Ocean Spray®)	68	250 mL	24
Gatorade	78	250 mL	12
Orange juice, unsweetened	50	250 mL	12
Tomato juice, canned	38	250 mL	4
BREAKFAST CEREALS AND RELATED PRODUCTS			
All-Bran®, average	55	30	12
Coco Pops®, average	77	30	20
Cornflakes®, average	93	30	23
Cream of Wheat® (Nabisco)	66	250	17
Cream of Wheat®, Instant (Nabisco)	74	250	22
Grapenuts, average	75	30	16
Muesli, average	66	30	16
Oatmeal, average	55	250	13
Instant oatmeal, average	83	250	30
Puffed wheat, average	80	30	17
Raisin Bran® (Kellogg's)	61	30	12
Special K® (Kellogg's)	69	30	14
GRAINS			
Pearled barley, average	28	150	12
Sweet corn on the cob, average	60	150	20
Couscous, average	65	150	9
Quinoa	53	150	13
White rice, average	73 ± 4	150	43
Quick cooking white basmati	67	150	28
Brown rice, average	68 ± 4	150	16
Converted, white rice (Uncle Ben's®)	38	150	14
Whole wheat kernels, average	30	50	11
Bulgur, average	48	150	12

COOKIES AND CRACKERS

Graham crackers	74	25	14
Vanilla wafers	77	25	14
Shortbread	64	25	10
Rice cakes, average	82	25	17
Rye crisps, average	64	25	11
Soda crackers	74	25	12

DAIRY PRODUCTS AND ALTERNATIVES

Ice cream, regular	57	50	6
Ice cream, premium	38	50	3
Milk, full fat	41	250 mL	5
Milk, skim	32	250 mL	4
Reduced-fat yogurt with fruit, average	33	200	11

FRUITS

Apple, average	39	120	6
Banana, ripe	62	120	16
Dates, dried	42	60	18
Grapefruit	25	120	3
Grapes, average	59	120	11
Orange, average	40	120	4
Peach, average	42	120	5
Peach, canned in light syrup	40	120	5
Pear, average	38	120	4
Pear, canned in pear juice	43	120	5
Prunes, pitted	29	60	10
Raisins	64	60	28
Watermelon	72	120	4

BEANS AND NUTS

Baked beans, average	40	150	6
Blackeye peas, average	33	150	10
Black beans	30	150	7
Chickpeas, average	10	150	3
Chickpeas, canned in brine	38	150	9
Navy beans, average	31	150	9

Kidney beans, average	29	150	7
Lentils, average	29	150	5
Soy beans, average	15	150	1
Cashews, salted	27	50	3
Peanuts, average	7	50	0
PASTA and NOODLES			
Fettucini, average	32	180	15
Macaroni, average	47	180	23
Macaroni and Cheese (Kraft)	64	180	32
Spaghetti, white, boiled, average	46	180	22
Spaghetti, white, boiled 20 min, average	58	180	26
Spaghetti, wholemeal, boiled, average	42	180	17
SNACK FOODS			
Corn chips, plain, salted, average	42	50	11
Fruit Roll-Ups®	99	30	24
M & M's®, peanut	33	30	6
Microwave popcorn, plain, average	55	20	6
Potato chips, average	51	50	12
Pretzels, oven-baked	83	30	16
Snickers Bar®	51	60	18
VEGETABLES			
Green peas, average	51	80	4
Carrots, average	35	80	2
Parsnips	52	80	4
Baked russet potato, average	111	150	33
Boiled white potato, average	82	150	21
Instant mashed potato, average	87	150	17
Sweet potato, average	70	150	22
Yam, average	54	150	20

MISCELLANEOUS			
Hummus (chickpea salad dip)	6	30	0
Chicken nuggets, frozen, reheated in microwave oven 5 min	46	100	7
Pizza, plain baked dough, served with parmesan cheese and tomato sauce	80	100	22
Pizza, Super Supreme (Pizza Hut)	36	100	9
Honey, average	61	25	12

Reprinted from Harvard Health Publications, Harvard Medical School.

Eliminating Gluten, Dairy, and Soy: Because gluten, dairy, and soy cause inflammatory responses in your body, it is my personal and professional opinion that they should be eliminated completely from the diets of those with any autoimmune condition. The easiest way to do this would be to look at the foods recommended in an eating plan like the paleo diet. (Numerous books and articles about this are available online.) This dietary adjustment can be extremely beneficial for people with diabetes.

Staying Away from Artificial Sweeteners: Even though some people refer to white sugar as *white death*—a term used by my esteemed colleague, Dr. Michael Johnson—artificial sweeteners, like aspartame (most commonly sold under the brand name, *NutraSweet*), are absolutely horrendous as well. But once it is heated, as it is once ingested—aspartame can turn into a formaldehyde-like substance, which can accumulate around your brain. It has been shown to be a potential cancer-causing or carcinogenic agent.

If you're trying to avoid sugar, don't jump to artificial sweeteners just because you want something sweet in your coffee or food. Instead, try small amounts of natural sweeteners like:

- Stevia
- Agave
- Raw, unprocessed honey
- Coconut sugar
- Blackstrap molasses
- Pure maple syrup (*not* maple-flavored corn syrup)

When it comes to sweeteners, a little goes a long way.

Other flavorings I recommend including in your diet are:

- Cinnamon (*not* cinnamon-sugar, just pure ground cinnamon)
- Apple cider vinegar (ACV)

Try to stay away from:

- Trans fats (can be carcinogenic)
- Starches
- Excessive alcohol (which can cause your blood sugar level to rise and then drop dramatically)

Case Study:

Myasthenia Gravis Case: Dr. Ed Beyer, DC, Board-Eligible Chiropractic Neurologist (Chicago, Illinois)

Rita is a fifty-nine-year-old city supervisor for the city of Chicago who came into my office with the chief complaints of severe fatigue, double vision, brain fog, constipation, and vertigo.

She mentioned in her history that she could not walk up a flight of stairs without extreme fatigue that would last for up to an hour. She had been diagnosed with an autoimmune disease known as *myasthenia gravis*. This is a disease in which the immune system is mistakenly attacking the receptor sites for the neurotransmitter called *acetylcholine*. This neurotransmitter plays an important role in our voluntary muscle contractions and in our digestive function.

Rita was also a Type 2 diabetic for which she was on two different medications: metformin and Levemir. From a functional medicine approach, we ran several specific lab tests trying to discover what was triggering Rita's immune system to attack parts of her own body. The blood test revealed that her glycosylated hemoglobin, which is a ninety-day blood sugar marker, was very high: a 9.9 despite her blood sugar medication.

Elevated blood sugar is widely accepted in scientific literature as an autoimmune trigger. Other triggers to her condition were also discussed. She had a sensitivity to gluten and corn. Stool analysis showed a gut infection of *helicobacter pylori* and a yeast infection as well.

The bloodwork also showed she had an autoimmune condition known as *Hashimotos' thyroiditis* affecting her thyroid.

An organic acids test showed very poor mitochondrial function (the mitochodria are the powerhouses of our cells) due to low glutathione, B vitamins, and CoQ10 status. Her vitamin D levels were very low as well. Vitamin D is very important for proper immune function.

We placed Rita on a paleo-type diet excluding all types of grains and dairy. We initially put her on a gut detoxification program with known botanicals to kill the guy infections. We included supplements that would lower her blood sugar, such as activated B vitamins, magnesium, chromium, alpha-lipoic acid, inositol, and gymnema sylvestre. We restricted high complex carbohydrates.

We also added Vitamin D, glutathione, and CoQ10. Neurologically, we gave her exercise to stimulate her lower brainstem and vagus nerve. This improved her gut function and constipation. Within weeks, Rita's fatigue was lifting and she could do things she hadn't done in years.

After three months, she was exercising thirty minutes per day, lost thirty pounds and was having regular bowel movements. Within six months she was off her type 2 diabetes medications. In tears she proclaimed to me that she had finally gotten her life back.

2

Fibromyalgia

MISCONCEPTIONS, CHARACTERIZATIONS, AND PRE-DISPOSITIONS

One of the biggest misconceptions about fibromyalgia is that it is not a real medical problem. Over the last few years, this has been the topic of much conversation among doctors.

Is Fibromyalgia Real?

It used to be that when doctors, whether MDs, DOs, DCs, or even PTs, could not figure out what was wrong with a patient, they would use fibromyalgia as a default. As such, since they could not come up with specific symptomatology and consistent, reproduceable treatment protocols, it became evident to many in the healthcare field that fibromyalgia was not a REAL condition.

Later, we began to see a slight shift as the number of people with symptoms grew.

From here, we started to see some diagnostic features of fibromyalgia, such as multiple tender points and fatigue for a minimum of a three-month period; if you did not meet those criteria, then you did not suffer from fibromyalgia.

We know now that this is truly not the case, as all individuals who suffer from fibromyalgia present with a multitude of symptomatology. But the one true constant that is across the board with all autoimmune conditions is inflammation.

Until recently, that was the conventional medical diagnosis of fibromyalgia. Unless you had those specific symptoms, many medical doctors were not ready to give the diagnosis.

An article in *Neurology Now*:

> *Researchers at the University of Michigan in Ann Arbor have found that patients with fibromyalgia have what's called a "hyperexcitable" nervous system. In other words, pain networks in their brains are more easily activated than people who don't have fibromyalgia. Other researchers have also found impairments in a specific brain region that helps to inhibit the body's response to pain among people with fibromyalgia. (Shaw, 2009)*

This research supports what I will be covering throughout this chapter — not just from a clinical point of view for my colleagues to read, but using different opinions to form a well-rounded resource for you to relate to personally.

What Is Fibromyalgia, and How Do You Get It?

Fibromyalgia is a chronic condition characterized by:

- Generalized aches and pains
- Fatigue
- Difficulty sleeping
- Sensitivities
- Chronic headaches

Other symptoms include:

- Dizziness
- Lightheadedness
- Menstrual cramping
- Jaw pain
- Restless leg syndrome
- Temporal mandibular joint (TMJ) pain

Scientists are now starting to realize that these symptoms are not caused by just a bone disease or a widespread pain condition but by an actual major problem associated with the brain and the nervous system. New research suggests that imbalances in the nervous system amplify normal sensations, making them even more painful. If you are super-sensitive to pain, there's a very good possibility that there is a genetic component.

An article in the *Journal of Neuroscience* concisely defines it:

Fibromyalgia is an intractable widespread pain disorder that is most frequently diagnosed in women. It has traditionally been classified as either a musculoskeletal disease or a psychological disorder. Accumulating evidence now suggests that fibromyalgia may be associated with CNS [central nervous system] dysfunction. (Kuchinad et al., 2007)

Some of the most up-to-date healthcare facilities in the United States, such as the Mayo Clinic, are saying that it's frustrating to treat people with fibromyalgia because the conventional treatment approaches aren't effective. They just don't work.

In the United States, an estimated *ten million* people are suffering from this disorder. That's a third of the population of Canada!

With ten million people suffering—and getting no relief— where can you go for answers?

These days, people are turning to television programs and websites for more information.

According to surgeon, author, and television personality, Dr. Mehmet Oz (2009):

- Even though it's classified as a musculoskeletal system disease, the condition is now seen as a central nervous system problem.

- The Western medical approach for a formal diagnosis didn't exist until 1990; Western medicine is slow to accept fibromyalgia and is way behind in its work.

- This is an area in which patients should take a serious look at alternative approaches.

When a popular mainstream health figure like Dr. Oz tells you to seek alternative approaches, it's clear that the conventional approach has not been working properly.

Dr. Andrew Weil—a medical doctor who runs an integrative medicine practice in Arizona—is one of the world's foremost authorities on complementary and alternative medicine. His research, showing that super-sensitive pain does appear to be genetic, indicates that fibromyalgia runs in families, and researchers have identified one particular gene that is believed to be involved in the syndrome (Weil, 2016).

Fibromyalgia patients also have higher than normal levels of the neuropeptide *substance P (SP)*, which is involved in the communication of signals to the brain. This predisposition is the condition's autoimmune component.

You could think of it like turning on a light.

1. You're born with the gene.
2. The gene is expressed.

3. You begin to display the symptoms associated with fibromyalgia.

What Can You Do About Fibromyalgia?

This disease affects the metabolic system, central nervous system, and musculoskeletal system, resulting in a wide range of symptoms that are not just related to pain.

The full range of symptoms can include:

- Chronic pain
- Chronic fatigue
- Insomnia or sleep disturbances
- Brain fog
- Irritable bowel syndrome (IBS)
- Migraine or cluster headaches
- Loss of memory or impaired memory
- Skin sensitivity
- Anxiety
- Tinnitus (ringing in the ears)
- Dry mouth
- Dizziness

Rather than trying to cure fibromyalgia or treat its symptoms, my goal is to treat the patient as a whole. For the remainder of this chapter, I'm going to approach fibromyalgia in the same way that I treat patients in my office: from the metabolic side and from the neurologic side.

THE METABOLIC SIDE

Fibromyalgia can be caused by:

- Inflammation
- Toxins
- Decreased immune response

But what causes these things?

Acidity

The first cause of massive inflammation, toxicity, and decreased immune response is acidity. When your body is too acidic, you need to make it more alkaline in order to heal.

What does that mean?

Your body's level of acidity or alkalinity is measured on a *pH scale* of 0–14, with the normal range for the human body being between 6.4 and 7.0. If your body is more acidic (indicated by a pH above 7.0), then it will be more vulnerable to disease processes.

How do we test pH?

Determining your body's pH is a very simple process, using pH testing strips—just like the ones you may remember using when you learned about pH in school. You can get a vial of pH strips on the Internet or at your local drugstore for about ten dollars, and they will last you a few months.

The strips can be used to test your urine or saliva. Because your body is metabolizing food throughout the day, your first void of urine in the morning is the most viable source for getting an accurate indication of your body's pH.

What causes your body to become acidic?

Causes of acidity include:

- Heavy metals
- Dental infections
- Poor diet
- Toxins

My colleagues and I do a lot of additional testing to determine the source of your symptoms, so we can set your body on a path to proper healing. While very few doctors pay much attention to the parathyroid gland, it protects you from heavy metal exposure and maintains your body's calcium levels. It helps buffer your blood. If your parathyroid is not working, your blood will not be buffered, which will make your body too acidic.

When your body is acidic:

- It pulls minerals out of your bones and places them in your bloodstream to buffer your blood.

- You're more likely to have heavy metal toxicity, which promotes the production of free radicals.

- Your internal environment becomes a breeding ground for viruses and bacteria.

Think about trying to light a match. If you go outside when it's raining or extremely windy, the match won't light. You need to have the right environment in order for it to work.

It's the same with your body. If you give bacteria and viruses a breeding ground in which to multiply, they will love it. But if you make it difficult (like trying to light a match underwater), you won't allow them to multiply and continue to wreak havoc on your body.

If you've ever wondered why you're susceptible to getting colds and the flu, acidity in your body may be why.

Free Radicals and Excitotoxins

The second cause of inflammation, toxicity, and a lowered immune response is cell damage from free radicals and excitotoxins.

Free radicals (unstable and highly reactive molecular particles that are formed when weak chemical bonds are broken) can damage the mitochondrial DNA in your cells and are the precursors to cancer and other long-term health problems.

Excitotoxins (chemicals that overstimulate neuron receptors) can cause premature cell death when their action is prolonged.

Research shows that long before fibromyalgia is diagnosed, the affected individuals have had poor nutritional habits and have typically been exposed to toxic chemicals and heavy metals. This leads to the production of free radicals and excitotoxins.

Diets that include trans-fatty acids and hydrogenated oils can cause your body to produce free radicals, and many of the most popular types of foods — including Chinese food and diet soft drinks — contain excitotoxins like monosodium glutamate (MSG) and aspartame.

If you know that you're not eating as well as you could be, then maybe you've turned to dietary supplements to give you the nutrients that you've been missing.

But where do you go for your supplements?

Every day, patients tell me that they're buying supplements like *Centrum* or *One A Day* from stores like Costco or Walmart. They think that for three or four dollars, they are getting their daily regimen of vitamins and minerals, and that they don't need to take anything else because these supplements have everything they need.

Why would you spend extra money on supplements if you can get them at a low price from Costco?

Because poor quality supplements can actually cause problems.

Typically, lower-priced supplements from these types of stores include synthetic forms of nutrients rather than the natural forms, and synthetic nutrients can cause free radicals and excitotoxins in your body.

Another poor dietary choice is eating highly processed, enriched foods. Enriched breads, pastas, crackers, cereals, waffles, and pancake mixes have added ingredients that could cause inflammation in your body. When vitamin C with ascorbic acid is consumed with enriched foods, the iron in the enriched foods can cause the oxidation of the ascorbic acid, creating dehydroascorbic acid (DHA), a free radical that is very harmful to your brain's neurons.

Free radicals and excitotoxins can also be caused by exposure to toxic chemicals, including hormones in meat and dairy products as well as pesticides in fruits and vegetables. There's a big difference between getting organic fruits and vegetables from a small, local farm and buying them from a large organic producer that is situated near a farm that uses pesticides, which could result in cross contamination.

Organophosphates, which are the basis of many insecticides and herbicides, have been listed by the United States Environmental Protection Agency (EPA) as highly toxic to humans. They defeat the liver's ability to detoxify, which is a very important function for the healing of tissue. If you're a farmer and you suffer from fibromyalgia, take a look at the pesticides you've been using on your crops. They might be the cause of your problem.

Exposure to toxic environmental factors, such as cell phones, cell phone towers, and Wi-Fi, can also cause free radicals and excitotoxins, as can exposure to heavy metals from mercury in amalgam dental fillings and nickel in dental crowns. Having two dissimilar metals in a saline solution will make a battery, which can cause mercury to leach out of the amalgams much faster. This could be happening in your mouth. If you've had dental amalgams and crowns sitting in your mouth for years, they could be a source of mercury contamination. Mercury can also be found in pest-control fumigants that are used in buildings.

Aluminum in antiperspirants is also a problem.

Did you ever wonder why it's called an *anti*perspirant?

How does it stop you from perspiring?

If you're using an antiperspirant as opposed to an all-natural deodorant, you will find that it contains aluminum. Aluminum gets into your pores and clogs them up so you can't perspire anymore. That's what an antiperspirant does; it puts metal into your body so you can't perspire. You definitely want to avoid that. One of the first things I tell people with fibromyalgia is to get rid of their antiperspirant and use a natural deodorant.

If you are suffering from fibromyalgia or any other disease, decreasing or eliminating your exposure to heavy metals and toxic synthetic chemicals can help you decrease some of the symptoms.

Infection

The third cause of inflammation, toxicity, and a lowered immune response is infection.

This can include:

- Dental infections
- Root canals
- Gut infections
- Parasites

- Viruses
- Bacterial Infections

While you may not want to think about things living in your body, there are trillions of bacteria in your gut alone.

Yes, *trillions*.

You also have small animals, called *parasites*, living in your body at all times. The most common parasites that infest humans are pinworms, roundworms, hookworms, and tapeworms. There are smaller parasites such as flukes, protozoa, amoebae, and fungi. The larger parasites can cause a lot of problems, particularly in your kidneys, liver, and gallbladder.

SIBO, or *Small Intestinal Bacterial Overgrowth*, occurs when bacteria from the colon move or migrate into the small intestine. Gases (hydrogen and methane) are produced by these bacteria, which cause a disruption in the digestive tract. This can lead to excess gas, bloating, and even diarrehea.

Helicobacter Pylori, or *H. Pylori*, is a parasitic infection that we call a "gram-negative bacteria," which can cause problems in the digestive system. Due to their physical makeup and corkscrew-type shape, the bacteria really embed themselves into whatever they infect, such as the lining of the stomach. This can lead to ulcers and other secondary problems.

Hypochlorhydria and Methylation

Being born with a gene that predisposes you to a particular disease — like multiple sclerosis (MS), Parkinson's, Alzheimer's, or cancer — does not necessarily mean that your body will express that gene and develop the condition.

So why — all of a sudden — would you start experiencing the symptoms of fibromyalgia?

What would cause your body to express that gene?

The gene can actually be passed on to you in either the turned-on or turned-off position, and what causes it to turn on are *depleted methyl groups*. When you have sufficient methyl groups, good genes — like tumor suppressor genes — are turned on, and the bad genes are turned off. When you have insufficient methyl groups (and bad genes), it can turn on *oncogenes*, the precursor to cancers, as well as turning off the tumor or cancer-supressor cells.

Methyl groups are needed for liver detoxification, regulation of protein function, and other important biological processes. They are important for normal cell replication, especially at the level of your DNA. In addition to fibromyalgia and cancer, inadequate methylation capacity can lead to birth defects, depression, cognitive decline, and autism.

What helps to create methyl groups?

Hydrochloric acid.

This is why it's vital to have the right amount of stomach acid.

Remember when I told you that 80 percent of your immune system is in your gut?

One of the biggest problems I see with fibromyalgia patients is hypochlorhydria, which means a lack of hydrochloric acid. Hydrochloric acid allows for the flow of your lymphatic system, and it's your primary methyl producer.

With the billions of dollars being spent on antacids every year, you'd think that a lack of antacids was causing people to have ulcers and acid reflux disease. But people aren't having these problems because they didn't take their TUMS® today. When there's not enough hydrochloric acid in your stomach, your lower esophageal sphincter doesn't close down, which causes hydrochloric acid to come up, giving you that heartburn feeling.

If you don't have the right amount of hydrochloric acid, the food you eat will rot in your stomach, and your body won't receive the proper nutrients from it. No matter what supplements you're taking, if your body is not able to absorb nutrients from food, you will never get better. Only when your stomach has enough hydrochloric acid will your gut be able to heal.

How do we determine if you have hypochlorhydria?

We test your blood for:

- Total protein
- Blood urea nitrogen (BUN)
- Cryoglobulins
- Phosphorus
- Calcium
- Creatinine

Immune System Support

As described in the introduction of this book, an autoimmune disease occurs when your immune system attacks itself.

How do you stop your immune system from attacking your body?

You need to:

- Decrease inflammation
- Detoxify your body
- Build up your immune system

Your immune system is made up of T helper cells know as T_h1 and T_h2. T_h1 cells are the destroyers of foreign invaders, and T_h2

cells are the antibodies that remember the invaders. To function properly, these two types of helper cells must be in balance.

Imagine this scenario:

- A friend of yours is suffering from cancer.

- Your friend hears from another friend that taking maitake (a type of mushroom) will help them.

Is this true?

Well, that depends on whether their immune system is dominant in T_h1 or in T_h2. If T_h1 is dominant, then their T_h2 will need to be supported, and if T_h2 is dominant, then their T_h1 will need to be supported.

The following supplements can be used to support immune system balance.

For T_h1 support:

- Vitamin A
- Vitamin C
- Zinc
- Astragalus
- Echinacea
- Licorice
- Lemon balm
- Maitake
- Garlic

For T_h2 support:

- Pine bark extract
- Green tea extract
- Grapeseed extract
- Resveratrol

- Pycnogenol
- Lycopene
- Caffeine

How do you determine which type of T helper cell is more dominant in you?

You can find out by taking a blood test.

THE NEUROLOGIC SIDE

The neurologic side of fibromyalgia is the central nervous system component — the brain component.

You may be thinking:

I don't have a brain tumor. There's nothing wrong with my brain.

What does my brain have to do with my pain?

In order to answer this question, it's important to understand what normal brain function is.

Brain Function and Stress

Just as your brain has a right side and a left side, there are also two sides to your *cerebellum*, which is an extremely important part of your lower brain that governs balance and coordination, controls your postural back movements, and coordinates your eye movements. As long as your cerebellum is receiving the proper amount of nerve input, there will be sufficient nerve input to your brain's frontal lobes, allowing them to send enough nerve input to your lower brainstem to keep your *mesencephalon* (midbrain) firing properly. In functional neurology, we refer to this process as *frequency of firing*.

Various types of chemical, physical, and emotional stress can cause an increase in the brain's frequency of firing. If one side of your cerebellum isn't receiving the proper amount of nerve input, then it can't send the proper amount of nerve input to your frontal lobe, and your frontal lobe then can't send the proper amount of input to your brainstem to keep your mesencephalon from over-firing.

Having an overactive mesencephalon can cause you to experience things like:

- Chronic pain
- Chronic fatigue
- Insomnia
- Light sensitivity
- Migraine headaches
- Blurred vision
- Constipation
- Diarrhea
- Irritable bowel syndrome (IBS)
- Heart palpitations
- Urinary tract infections
- High blood pressure
- Brain fog

Do these symptoms look familiar?

They look like the symptoms of fibromyalgia, don't they?

If your midbrain is over-firing, a multitude of symptoms express themselves.

How does an over-firing midbrain cause you to experience these symptoms?

Your midbrain houses some very important functions. For example, the origins of your eye function are housed in your midbrain. Your *oculomotor nerve*, also known as your third cranial nerve, regulates the dilation or constriction of your pupils. If your pupils are not constricting and too much light is going into your eyes, then you're going to become light sensitive.

What about migraines?

While the brain itself doesn't have any pain receptors (you could actually be awake during brain surgery and not feel a thing), the mesh that surrounds the brain does. When your midbrain is over-firing, the blood vessels in your brain dilate and the nerve mesh around the blood vessels becomes irritated. That's what migraine pain is.

If your midbrain is over-firing, the brain's medulla (located in the brainstem) is not receiving proper stimulation. This can affect your vagus nerve (your tenth cranial nerve), which interacts with your digestive tract, and can cause you to have constipation or diarrhea, or it can inhibit urination, causing a buildup that can lead to urinary tract infections.

Does it surprise you to learn that your brain can cause urinary tract infections?

While we may have a tendency to think of illness as localized, having a problem in a specific area doesn't mean that the problem's cause is in that same area.

Another system that can be affected by an over-firing midbrain is your body's regulator of wakefulness, the *mesencephalic reticular activating system* (RAS). This can lead to either insomnia or fatigue, depending on when the over-firing is occurring

- If the highest firing rate is at 3:00 a.m., it can to lead to insomnia.

- If the lowest firing rate is at 3:00 p.m., it can lead to fatigue.

What if that over-firing midbrain is sending messages down your spinal cord?

It can send messages to the electrical conduction system of your heart, such as your sinoatrial (SA) node and your atrioventricular (AV) node, causing your heart rate to speed up, or it can send messages to your adrenal glands.

Your adrenal glands are extremely important. They sit right above your kidneys, and they are your stress glands—they are affected by emotional, environmental, and physical stress. When your adrenals are stressed, hormones like epinephrine (adrenaline) and norepinephrine are released into your bloodstream, thereby stimulating your type C (slower) nociceptive (pain-sensing) nerve fibers. This process can cause the chronic pain that is associated with fibromyalgia, and the chronic pain can then cause fatigue due to sleep loss.

When you're under emotional stress, your brain's hypothalamus produces corticotropin-releasing factor (CRF), which stimulates your pituitary to release adrenocorticotropic hormone (ACTH), causing your adrenal medulla to release cortisol. Cortisol is toxic to your brain. When you have too much cortisol in your system, you experience problems focusing known as *fibro fog*.

Neurologic Treatment

Fibromyalgia itself does not get better on its own. The longer you have fibromyalgia, the more and faster your brain dies. The *Journal of Neuroscience* reports that McGill University Center for Research on Pain, located in Montreal, Quebec, has found that the longer the individual has had fibromyalgia, the greater the grey matter loss, with each year of having fibromyalgia being equivalent to 9.5 times the loss in normal aging. In addition, it is estimated that 30 to 60 percent of patients diagnosed with fibromyalgia become disabled to the degree that they can't remain gainfully employed, and that's with the myriad of medications they've already been prescribed (Kuchinad, et al., 2007).

How can we do things differently to help people get better?

From a brain-based perspective, we would look at your results from all the testing mentioned in the metabolic section, and then we'd develop a specific treatment plan to target any affected areas in your cerebellum and midbrain.

How do we treat the brain?

In order to function properly, the cerebellum and the midbrain require two things:

1. Fuel
2. Activation

For these two parts of your brain, fuel comes in the form of:

- Glucose
- Oxygen

The previously mentioned ketones are an alternative source.

Just as a lack of glucose can make you hypoglycemic, a lack of oxygen can make your brain shut down. When the brain is deprived of oxygen for a long enough period of time, the result is brain death.

Each year after age twenty-five, through a process called *oxidative phosphorylation* (OXPHOS), the body loses 1 percent of its ability to utilize oxygen. The lack of oxygen in your body will cause biological oxidation, which can damage your cells.

Increasing the amount of oxygen that goes into your brain allows your tissues to heal faster.

How do we do that?

Exercise With Oxygen Therapy

One of the most effective ways to increase oxygen to your brain is by using exercise with oxygen therapy.

In my office, we use a combination of:

- An oxygen concentrator—a machine that takes 90 percent of the oxygen out of the air and concentrates it into a cannula (breathing tube)

- An upper-body ergometer (UBE), which requires you to churn handles much in the same way a bicycle requires you to pedal with your feet

The UBE is one of the best types of exercise for this purpose because the closer we get to your brain, the more receptors there are, and it's much more powerful and effective to stimulate the brain where there are more receptors than where there are fewer.

Vibration and Manipulation

Vibration and manipulation are very good methods for stimulating your brain. Your mechanoreceptors (the receptors in your body that respond to pressure) are fired by the quick movement of your joints during chiropractic adjustment. Adjustments also activate your nervous system's large-diameter afferent fibers.

Your large-diameter afferents serve two functions:

1. To bring information to the back part of your spinal cord
2. To inhibit pain

Along these pathways, information travels very quickly—about 275 miles per hour. If the pathways aren't intact, you will lose your inhibition to pain, and you'll lose your ability to sense light touch and vibration, so it's very important for us to make sure that these large-diameter afferents are functioning properly.

PNRT and Auditory Stimulation

As mentioned in the diabetes chapter, besides adjustments or joint manipulation, one of the best ways to stimulate your large-diameter afferents is through Peripheral Neuropathy Rehabilitation Therapy (PNRT).

Another method is auditory stimulation. For this, we might perform a *warm caloric*—a simple, yet powerful, process in which we use a large syringe to inject warm, soapy water into your ear, and once the water hits your eardrum, it flows back out again. We do this to stimulate your *vestibulocochlear nerve* (your eighth cranial nerve), which then sends a signal to your cerebellum.

(I learned this treatment from Dr. Ted Carrick, one of the world's foremost authorities on chiropractic neurology, who was responsible for helping the professional hockey player, Sidney Crosby, get back on the ice after multiple head injuries and concussion syndromes.)

Regardless of the specific methods used, it's important to remember that there is no cure-all treatment for fibromyalgia. There is no quick fix for this type of disease process. It's not just a matter of localized pain, and we're not just going to give you a pill and hope that your pain goes away. You need to understand that there are other factors involved. There is a metabolic component and a neurologic component, and only a consideration of both of these components will fully support your body's ability to heal.

Case Study:

Fibromyalgia Case: Dr. Michael Glickert, DC, Director of Clinic Operations for the Vanguard Clinic (St. Louis, Missouri)

Our clinic focuses on treating patients suffering with a variety of chronic conditions including autoimmune diseases. My favorite testimonial comes from my patient Jessica. Jessica had an autoimmune condition for decades and has suffered with fibromyalgia for over twenty years. She was fifty-one when she started care in our office, which means her symptoms started in her early thirties.

We met at a chamber of commerce luncheon and we talked about her diagnosis and symptoms. I told her we could most likely help her find some answers and she agreed to come in for a consultation and exam.

Jessica told me about the dozens of doctors that she had seen and all the medication that she's been recommended. She hated taking all the medication as the side effects were giving her a hard time. She is a co-owner of a small business and was only working three days a week. Some days, her pain was so bad that she couldn't even get out of bed.

We started aggressively with Jessica and she was an extremely compliant patient. She listened to everything that I recommended. She changed her diet; she took the recommended nutrition products; she did all of the home therapies I suggested.

She quickly started feeling better and within just a few weeks she was back to working five days a week. While we were both thrilled about her working a full week, what she told me after working with her for three months brought tears to my eyes.

She told me that at the age of forty-five, she and her husband stopped having sex because her pain "down there" was so bad. She had been to half-a-dozen specialists, including a vulva specialist. She tried creams, lotions, pills, and everything these specialists suggested she try. Nothing worked.

After three months of working with her she was once again having sex. She told me she couldn't believe that by cleaning up her diet, taking recommended nutrition and focusing on really getting healthy that she was once again able to have a sexual relationship with her husband. Needless to say, both she and her husband are extremely happy that we were able to help her.

3

Autoimmune Thyroid Disorders

Your thyroid is known as *the master switch* for your body. Think of it as the thermostat that will control how your body reacts to the environment.

How does this happen?

Let's begin with the brain. Your brain sends a signal through the hypothalamus to the pituitary gland. This connection, also known as the H-P or hypothalamic-pituitary axis, controls the amount of thyroid stimulating hormone or TSH, adrenal hormones, and many male and female hormones.

As TSH is released to the thyroid gland, TSH causes enzyme TPO to stimulate the release Of T_4 (93 percent) and T_3 (7 percent). These hormones ride the metaphoric taxicab of thyroid-binding globule (TBG). TBG (the taxicab) escorts T_3 to the liver, gut, and peripheral tissues, where the T_4 is transformed into the active form T_3, which then enters the cells via the cell receptor sites.

The following symptoms are associated with thyroid dysfunction:

- Fatigue
- Increase in weight gain, even with low-calorie diet

- Morning headaches that wear off as the day progresses
- Depression
- Constipation
- Overly sensitive to cold weather
- Poor circulation and numbness in hands and feet
- Muscle cramps while at rest
- Catch colds and other viral or bacterial problems easily with difficult recovery
- Wounds heal slowly
- Require excessive amount of sleep to function properly
- Chronic digestive problems (hypochlorhydria)
- Itchy, dry skin
- Dry or brittle hair
- Hair falls out easily
- Edema, especially facial (myxedema)
- Loss of outside portion of eyebrows

HASHIMOTO'S THYROIDITIS AND GRAVES' DISEASE

Dr. Hakaru Hashimoto (1881–1934) was a Japanese physician at the medical school of Kyushu University. In 1912, Dr. Hashimoto published a clinical paper in Germany that first outlined his research on autoimmune thyroid disease. Thus, the disease was named after him.

In 1912, he studied the cases of four women with enlarged thyroid glands that seemed to have changed into lymphoid tissue, or *struma lymphomatosa*. After thyroid surgery, the patients became hypothyroid.

Forty years after his studies, antithyroid antibodies were found in patients with this disorder. Hashimoto's is now recognized as one form of *autoimmune thyroiditis*. Another form is called *atrophic thyroiditis*. They are similar to each other in that they both have thyroid autoantibodies in serum. But the Hashimoto's includes the presence of a goiter, or goiter-like growth, and the atrophic condition does not.

Thyroid autoimmunity appears to be inheritable as a dominant trait. Doctors Colin Dayan and Gilbert Daniels, in a *New England Journal of Medicine* article, note that, "Up to 50 percent of the first-degree relatives of patients with chronic autoimmune thyroiditis have thyroid antibodies, apparently inherited as a dominant trait" (Dayan and Daniels, 1996).

Because thyroid autoimmunity is inheritable, it is likely that relatives will develop thyroid issues.

If you have Hashimoto's disease, your immune system attacks your thyroid gland for reasons researchers have yet to understand. It may be due to a genetic flaw. Other theories suggest a virus or bacterium may trigger the response. Still other possibilities are that a combination of factors, such as sex, age, and heredity, play a role in whether you develop this disorder.

While many of us may have heard that too low an iodine intake creates problems with the thyroid (one of the reasons it's added to many table salt brands), too much is correlated with thyroiditis. This is found most often in the United States and Japan, which have the highest intake of iodine.

The resulting inflammation from Hashimoto's leads to an underactive (*hypo-*) or sometimes overactive (*hyper-*) thyroid gland. This is the most common cause of hypothyroidism in the United States. It primarily affects middle-aged women, but it can also affect men, women of any age, and children. Right now in the United States, it's affecting approximately thirty million people. That is roughly the population of Canada.

Having another autoimmune disease, such as rheumatoid arthritis, diabetes, or lupus increases your risk of developing Hashimoto's disease.

Testing for Hashimoto's

How do you know if you have Hashimoto's thyroiditis?

What kind of testing is available?

We like to use a *thyroid peroxidase* or TPO test.

TPO is a thyroid enzyme involved in hormone production. If there are TPO antibodies in your blood, that could mean that you have thyroid autoimmunity, such as Hashimoto's or Graves' disease, and your body is calling for an attack of the TPO because it mistakes it for an unhealthy substance that must be eradicated.

THYROID FUNCTION AND PHYSIOLOGY

Did you know that every cell in your body has thyroid receptors?

Having thyroid receptors in every single cell in your body means that there are a lot of things to consider when we are looking at thyroid conditions.

You may be asking yourself:

Why doesn't my endocrinologist know this?

If I'm going to a specialist, like an endocrinologist, who specializes in the endocrine system (and a lot of them specialize in autoimmune disorders, specifically with the thyroid or with diabetes) *and if I'm also seeing an internal medicine specialist, why do they not know these additional tests or these additional therapies?*

While some physicians read medical journals, the overwhelming majority of them do not.

Why don't they?

They simply don't have the time. In our modern, insurance-mandated world, they're stuck looking at patients, one after another, and they really just don't have the time or the desire to research the most up-to-date treatments. They rely on what they learned in school—maybe fifteen, twenty, or thirty years ago. Quite simply, most of that is outdated.

When you're suffering from any kind of thyroid problem, you're suffering not just from the condition of the thyroid itself. Because there are thyroid receptors in every cell in your body, you're going to be suffering from a *web of physiological dysfunction*—a term coined by two of my esteemed colleagues, Dr. Andy Barlow and Dr. Michael Johnson. Nobody has just one problem. With thyroid issues, that's a physiological impossibility. When you seek care for your chief complaint, you could end up discovering that you have adrenal dysfunction, brain dysfunction, immune system imbalances, and hormone imbalances.

If you think you should take a pill for your thyroid problem, then you might want to ask yourself:

How could there possibly be a pill for this?

They don't make a pill that cures everything.

When you're dealing with a web of physiological dysfunction, you can't just take one pill, like Synthroid, to fix it.

It Starts With Your Brain

When it comes to the thyroid, your brain is extremely important. Your brain controls every function in your body. It sends electrical signals down your spinal cord and out to every single organ in your body. Whether it's your eyes, your stomach, your lungs, your pancreas, or your thyroid, everything has a nerve going to it, and that nerve has to work. That means that if your brain is malfunctioning, it can affect every part of your anatomy.

Your Frontal Lobe: The frontal lobe of the brain houses our executive function — decision-making, problem solving, and planning, as well as many other cognitive functions.

Have you noticed personality changes, such as depression, anxiety, or irritability?

These are all components of your frontal lobe.

Your Hippocampus: The hippocampus is one of the places where you store long-term and emotional memory. Some memory problems, such as the creation of new memories, are dependent upon the health of the hippocampus.

Your Parietal Lobe: This is where all sensory input fires into your brain. Any information that you get from touching things, these sensory-information pathways go to the parietal lobe. If the parietal lobe starts to short-circuit, then you're going to have pain, numbness, and tingling throughout your body.

How many pills are there to fix your parietal lobe?

None!

What if you have short-term memory loss?

How many pills are there to fix your short-term memory bank?

None!

Thyroid Metabolism

In order to improve your health, we have to understand how your thyroid is actually functioning.

In normal thyroid metabolism, your hypothalamus, located at the base of your brain, sends thyroid-releasing hormone (TRH) to your pituitary gland. Your pituitary gland releases thyroid-stimulating hormone (TSH) to your thyroid gland. This stimulates your thyroid peroxidase activity to use iodine to create thyroxine (T_4) and triiodothyronine (T_3) antibodies.

The majority of your thyroid hormones, 93 percent, are T_4, which is the inactive form. Only 7 percent are the active form, the ones your body actually uses. When you go to your doctor for standard thyroid testing, they'll test your T_3, but they may not check your T_4.

So what happens to all the T_4?

Thyroid Hormone Conversion

Sixty percent of your T_4 is converted to T_3 in your liver. Twenty percent goes to reverse T_3, which is the inactive form, 20 percent is converted to T_3S, which is inactive, and the remaining T_4 is converted to T_3 in your peripheral tissues. When you have the T_3, that is converted to active T_3 in your gastrointestinal tract, or your gut, and that leads to the active form of T_3.

What does all this mean?

It means that if you only relied on testing for T_3, you would only be getting 7 percent of the active form of TSH. You have to make sure that your liver and your gut are functioning properly because if those two are not functioning properly, then your thyroid may not be functioning properly.

How does this conversion take place?

My friend and esteemed colleague, Dr. Andy Barlow, came up with a great analogy.

Think of T_4 as a coffee bean and T_3 as the coffee that's been ground into a usable form. In order to put it into your coffee machine, you have to first put that coffee bean into a coffee mill and process it so that it's usable.

For the most part, that's your liver's job. If your liver doesn't process that T_4, you don't have access to 93 percent of what's available. You just can't use it.

If all you're doing is testing the T_3 and supplementing with Synthroid, you're never going to get better.

Gut Function and Stomach Acid

If 80 percent of your immune system is in your gut, and you have poor gut function, you're going to have problems not only with the gut, but with the gut-brain connection as well.

The father of medicine, Hippocrates, said, "Look to the gut. There you will find the origin of almost all human illnesses."

Anything that can cause an immune battle in your gut will trigger inflammation.

For example:

- Food sensitivities
- Chronic infections
- Bacterial infections
- Parasites
- Mold
- Fungus
- Yeast
- Viruses
- Undergrowth of good bacteria or normal flora

Poor gut function is almost always due to the following:

- Food sensitivities to things like gluten, casein, soy, egg protein, and yeast
- Gut infections or abnormal levels of healthy gut bacteria
- Stomach acid imbalances or leaky gut syndrome (more information on this is in the gastrointestinal disorder chapter)

If you don't have enough acid in your stomach to break down your food, then the food will simply rot in your stomach. If the food is rotting in your stomach, then you won't be getting the nutrients out of it, or out of the supplements that you're taking, because you won't have them in a usable form.

Blood Sugar, Brain Function, and Your Adrenals

Another thing you need to be aware of with any kind of thyroid problem is that blood sugar is the primary fuel source for your brain. Because oxygen is extremely important to brain function, and oxygen feeds on glucose, poor blood sugar regulation leads to poor brain function.

Your adrenal glands (the small glands that sit on top of your kidneys, described in the chapter on diabetes) also play a significant role in thyroid function when they release cortisol and other hormones in response to stress.

But what happens when cortisol goes up?

Cortisol is toxic to your brain. When cortisol is increased, your hippocampus, which is responsible for short-term memory, is affected. There's a direct correlation between the amount of cortisol and the decreased function of your adrenal glands.

The adrenal glands also release epinephrine and norepinephrine, which stimulate pain-fibers abnormally. If the adrenals are not functioning properly that can, in turn, affect the function of your thyroid.

Crosstalk

Did you know that your thyroid *talks* to other parts of your body?

It's what we call crosstalk.

Your thyroid talks to:

- Your immune system
- Your gut
- The rest of your endocrine system

What this means is that each of them affects the outcome of the other, back and forth, like a conversation.

Your *hypothalamus-to-pituitary axis* controls thyroid hormones, adrenal hormones, and cortisol regulation. It controls male and female hormones, like estrogen, progesterone, and testosterone. Consequently, a problem with one of these will lead to a problem with the rest.

Functional Lab Values

If you've been told by your doctor that your lab tests are normal, you might be thinking:

My doctor said there's nothing wrong with me, so why do I feel so lousy?

The answer is that they might not be running the proper tests, or they might be using traditional lab ranges, which are inaccurate. This type of testing uses bell curves, and the bell curves are based on unhealthy people.

Functional lab values are much more sensitive, and they help to reveal problems you might have if your standard lab tests are normal but you don't feel well. While standard tests have abnormal low values and abnormal high values, functional lab ranges are right in the middle.

TSH: The standard lab range for TSH is 0.3 to 5.7 milli-international units per liter (mIU/L). The functional range is 1.8 to 3.0 mIU/L. That's where you want to be. When interpreting functional test results, 4.2 is considered hypothyroid. In a standard lab range, that would show up as a normal test, but if you're at 4.2, then there's already a problem.

Typically, thyroid tests are ordered for TSH, which only shows the T_3 (active form) that your body uses. If you're lucky (or if you specifically ask your doctor for a *thyroid panel*), they might also test for T_4.

But what tests are you still missing?

You want to make sure that the following tests are included as well.

FTI: Free thyroxin index (FTI) is the amount of T_4 that is available.

FT$_4$: Free thyroxin (Free T_4 or FT_4) can be affected by the medications that you're taking.

T$_3$ Uptake: This will tell you how much of the T_3 is taken up by thyroxine-binding globulin (TBG).

FT$_3$: Free triiodothyronine (Free T_3 or FT_3) is the active thyroid hormone.

You also want to look at reverse T_3 (rT_3), thyroid peroxidase antibodies (TPO Ab) and thyroglobulin antibodies (TGB Ab) (specifically when you're dealing with autoimmune conditions like Hashimoto's), TSH antibodies (TSH Ab) (when you're dealing with Graves' disease), and TBG levels.

Here's the point:

If you want to see something that's normal, get out your lawn chair, bring it to Walmart, sit down, and watch all the unhealthy and overweight people going in and buying their groceries.

But if you want to make sure that you're getting the proper testing and that you're feeling well, you have to make sure you're asking for these specific tests. Otherwise, you're going to be like all of those people who are just going along from day to day, getting the same standard of care, not changing anything, and thinking that they're healthy simply because their lab tests came back normal.

TREATMENTS

Hashimoto's, which is a combination of hypo- and hyperthyroid, and Graves' disease, which is more hyperthyroid, are not typically just thyroid problems; they are immune system problems. Your immune system is mistakenly attacking TPO or TBG (in Hashimoto's) or TSH (in Graves' disease).

With immune problems, there is an imbalance in your immune system that needs to be addressed. To determine what that imbalance is, you need to go through the proper testing.

The standard medical approach is to do minimal testing, wait until the tissue destruction is really bad, and then squash your entire immune system with steroids. If that doesn't work, then you can take an anti-depressant and hope for the best. They're looking at symptom management, and not addressing the underlying metabolic causes.

Complications

What are some of the complications from thyroid problems?

If left untreated, an underactive thyroid gland caused by Hashimoto's can lead to a number of health problems.

Goiter: A goiter is an enlargement of the thyroid gland. Although generally not uncomfortable, a large goiter can affect your appearance and interfere with things like swallowing or, potentially, even breathing.

Heart Problems: If left untreated, hyper- or hypothyroidism can lead to an enlarged heart and, in rare cases, even heart failure.

Depression: Mental health issues, like depression, can occur early on in thyroid diseases, especially in Hashimoto's, and may become more severe over time.

Birth Defects: Babies born to women with untreated hypothyroidism due to Hashimoto's may have a higher risk of birth defects than babies born to healthy mothers. There is a link between hypothyroidism pregnancies and birth defects, such as cleft palate.

These are some of the complicating factors that go along with leaving not just thyroid conditions, but autoimmune thyroid conditions, untreated.

A Functional Approach

With a functional medicine approach, our aim is to:

- Remove all of your immune triggers.
- Remove your food sensitivities.
- Remove any infections.
- Stabilize your blood sugar levels.
- Reduce any inflammation.

We address:

- Adrenal dysfunction
- Hormone dysfunction
- Thyroid dysfunction
- Liver and gallbladder problems

The Neuro-Metabolic Approach

We take that one step further and look at the neuro-metabolic approach as well.

To get the best results, we have to modulate the immune system by:

- Using dietary modification and lifestyle changes

- Adding supplements based on lab findings specific to your body's needs

- Addressing neurological misfiring and brain dysfunction, using brain-based therapy

- Combining that with functional neurology and functional medicine in order to treat you as a whole person and not just a specific disease

Case Study:

Autoimmune Thyroid Case: Dr. R Joel Rosen D.C, DAAIM, CFMP, Boca Health Care Center (Boca Raton, Florida) www. bocahealthcarecenter

Roberta was searching on the Internet because she's had been having so much pain for the last couple of years. Normally a very alert, quick minded owner of a business, along with her widespread musculoskeletal pain, she was having more and more difficulty with concentration, gastro-intestinal pain, difficulty with walking, sleeping, and just performing her normal activities.

Roberta was very similar to other chronic condition sufferers, in that she had always felt that there was more going on with her health beside the consistent feedback that her primary doctor was telling her, that all her blood tests were normal.

After a thorough medical history that includes childhood experiences, any illnesses that she had suffered with, medications that she had been taking and for how long, past dental history, infections, dental amalgams, antibiotic use in her lifetime, chemical exposures, surgical and hospitalization history, occupational hazards, and family history, it became evident that Roberta's immune system had been overly compromised from a cumulative perspective.

As the investigation process continued, building a patient story based on the subjective facts that Roberta revealed, the next step was to evaluate her recent blood tests from a functional perspective. That is, not scrutinizing the laboratory findings in terms of a normal test but, rather, determining whether or not her tests results fall within a healthy range. In Roberta's case, although she did not have diagnosis of anemia, she was trending toward anemic tendencies, as her red blood cell count and hemoglobin were functionally low.

Roberta told me that her doctor had never mentioned anything of the sort, which had not surprised me. That is because from a laboratory perspective, Roberta's tests were determined to be "normal" (when compared to the average sick person). But when she was compared to the average healthy person (a functional range), Roberta fell outside the "optimal ranges."

Because her red blood cells were carrying less oxygen, they were, in effect, delivering less fuel to the cells of her body, which is necessary for energy production and proper function. Test by test, we determined that Roberta also suffered with dysglycemia, or unstable blood sugar levels, elevated cholesterol and LDLs, both suggestive of insulin resistance.

Not only were Roberta's cells not getting the optimal oxygen for cellular function, so too were they not getting optimal fuel, in the way of glucose. Double whammy.

The final straw for Roberta was the fact that she had positive Thyroid Peroxidase Antibodies, which means that Roberta's immune system was over-reacting and in effect attacking her thyroid.

From these test results alone, we certainly had our initial game plan. My first goal was to address Roberta's immune dysregulation.

Because it is estimated that up to 80 percent of our immune system is in our gastro-intestinal tract, and the fact that Roberta was having gastro-intestinal symptoms, we needed to:

1. Identify the state of her gut

2. Assess what foods she may have developed an intolerance/sensitivity to

3. Remove the offending foods

4. Repair any permeability that may have developed.

Since identifying these foods, removing them from Roberta's diet, embarking on an intestinal repair protocol, and subsequently stabilizing Roberta's blood sugar levels, aiding with digestive secretions, Roberta has undergone a 180-degree turn.

Her red blood cell and hemoglobin levels are elevated and now within an optimal functional range, her blood sugar levels are optimized, her cholesterol levels have lowered, her thyroid antibodies have reduced, and, to boot, she has lost fifteen pounds in six weeks. She is more focused, more energetic, and experiencing less pain.

It sounds like an all-around great story, doesn't it?

However, I would like to add, not all chronic cases respond this way, this fast. That is because of the varying degrees of toxic exposure and immune compromise the chronic condition sufferer may have. Heavy metal toxicity, mercuries, mold exposures, multiple autoimmunities, hormonal imbalance . . . ALL must be addressed and held at bay before a complete recovery can be established.

4

Gastrointestinal Disorders

INTESTINAL FORTITUDE

The *gut* is a catch-all term for your gastrointestinal organs:

- Stomach
- Large intestine
- Small intestine
- Colon
- Everything else in your intestinal tract

Gut function, or *intestinal fortitude*, is extremely important to your health.

Conditions resulting from intestinal tract problems include:

- Irritable bowel syndrome (IBS)
- Celiac disease
- Ulcerative colitis
- Crohn's disease

This chapter will address the causes and specific nature of each of these problems, and what can be done about them.

Your Body's Screen Door

Traditionally, it was thought that the primary function of the gastrointestinal tract was to limit the digestion and absorption of nutrients, electrolytes, and water and to maintain a balance, or homeostasis. A better analysis of the anatomy and function of the gastrointestinal tract suggests that an extremely important function of this organ is to regulate the trafficking of *micromolecules* (smaller molecules) or *macromolecules* (larger molecules) between environments and the host through a barrier system that acts kind of like a screen door.

Think about how a screen door works in your house. It filters large things out. It doesn't allow bugs or birds to come into your house, but it does allow small particles, which don't cause much of a problem, to come through. If you allowed the large things to get through, it would really cause disequilibrium in your house.

Now, think of your body as having a screen door—a barrier system that stops major particles from getting in and causing problems. When your body's intestinal barrier isn't functioning properly, the irritation to your system can result in the development of autoimmunity and nervous system abnormalities.

Some of the factors that can affect your mucosal immune system, resulting in a dysfunction of your body's intestinal barrier, include:

- Diet
- Protein
- Peptides
- Antibodies
- Drugs
- Physical stress

- Infections
- Cytokines
- Neurotransmitters
- Enzymes

These things can start to break down the tight junctions that are naturally keeping everything locked into your gut. This causes an increase in *permeability* — the ability for things to get through these junctions. When the lining of your intestines becomes more permeable, allowing large molecules like food particles to permeate the system and wreak havoc on your immune system, we call this *leaky gut syndrome*.

A dysfunction of your intestinal barrier can lead to food allergies and intolerance of specific foods, which can lead to immune system abnormalities and, eventually, autoimmunity. If you developed allergies as a result of being exposed to multiple infections and medications as a child, and then even more drugs were used to combat those allergies, this could lead to autoimmune problems, like ulcerative colitis, rheumatoid arthritis, or diabetes.

Irritable Bowel Syndrome (IBS)

Irritable bowel syndrome has multiple and varied symptoms, and is generally considered to be a wastebasket diagnosis — meaning that because they cannot pinpoint a diagnosis, many doctors will just call a condition IBS by default. With IBS, even though your digestive tract may appear normal in imaging studies, it doesn't function properly. The rhythm of the muscles pushing food through your intestines fluctuates between extremely high and extremely low. These extremes cause you to have pain that comes and goes. Due to heightened sensitivity, you could experience bloating and swelling as well.

A lot of people who suffer from IBS also suffer from autoimmune disease. They have problems with constipation, diarrhea, or both. Repairing the gut is the most important thing you can do for these problems.

CELIAC DISEASE

Celiac disease, or *celiac sprue*, is an inherited autoimmune condition that attacks mainly the small intestine and is triggered by an increased sensitivity to gluten. Sprue is a general term referring to decreased absorption of the intestinal mucosa, which can be caused by the toxic effects of gluten on your digestive system. Gluten can damage or destroy the small, fingerlike projections, called *villi*, or the even smaller ones, called *microvilli*, allowing your absorption of proteins and carbohydrates to be diminished or impaired.

Once this process starts, it can lead to damage in other areas of your body, including your brain. Celiac disease is the only autoimmune disease that is actively started with a poor reaction to *gliadin*, the amino acid in gluten. While we do see an increased sensitivity to gluten in all autoimmune diseases, with celiac disease there's a direct correlation: it's a causative agent. When gliadin does not get completely absorbed, it causes an immune reaction that irritates or destroys the mucosal lining of your intestines.

Symptoms associated with celiac disease can include:

- Gas
- Bloating
- Cramps
- Chronic diarrhea
- Vomiting
- Liver dysfunction

- Infertility
- Anemia
- Weight loss
- Fatigue
- Joint pain
- Anxiety
- Depression

This disease affects nearly two million people in the United States — with 60 percent of those being children and 40 percent adults — and the process can be occurring without you even knowing it. You may be totally symptom free, but as it continues to progress and get worse, it will cause increased problems in your intestinal tract. By the time you start to feel it, there will already have been a lot of damage done, making it difficult to manage.

Specific testing for celiac disease can include:

- Serological testing and bloodwork
- CBC with an iron panel
- Erythrocyte sedimentation rate (ESR)
- Vitamin D levels
- Homocysteine

The following tests will give you a better overall picture of your condition:

- Thyroid panel
- Adrenal stress index
- Food sensitivity testing

When gluten is eliminated from your diet, you will see an improvement of symptoms. If you have any degree of celiac disease, it is essential for you to be gluten free.

ULCERATIVE COLITIS

Ulcerative colitis is an autoimmune disorder that attacks mostly the large intestine, also known as the bowel or colon. As the lining of your colon becomes inflamed, it starts to form ulcers.

Symptoms associated with ulcerative colitis include:

- Fatigue
- Loss of appetite
- Fever
- Diarrhea
- Anemia

In addition to bowel problems, you may also experience:

- Arthritis
- Rashes
- Skin disorders (thick or painful red areas on your skin)

Ulcerative colitis affects only six out of every one hundred thousand people, and the diagnosis generally occurs before the age of thirty. It is mainly confined to Jewish populations of eastern European descent. If you have a family history of ulcerative colitis, then you're at a much higher risk, particularly if you have a parent, sibling, or child with the disease.

To obtain a definitive diagnosis, standard gastrointestinal testing is usually accompanied by a colonoscopy.

Conventional treatments may include:

- Antibiotics
- Corticosteroids
- Immunosuppressive agents
- Immunomodulators

Because of the increase in ulcerations of the areas that it affects, ulcerative colitis can be totally debilitating.

Complications associated with ulcerative colitis include:

- Severe bleeding
- Perforations in the colon
- Osteoporosis
- Kidney stones
- Dehydration
- Increased risk of colon cancer

CROHN'S DISEASE

Crohn's disease, first identified in 1932 by Dr. Burrill B. Crohn, is an inflammation of the gastrointestinal tract. Originally called *terminal ileitis* for the specific area in the small intestine where the terminal ileum and the colon meet (the site most commonly affected), the word "terminal" scared patients because it gave them the impression that the disease was fatal.

The inflammation from Crohn's disease can affect different levels of the bowel wall and can cause symptoms similar to other intestinal disorders, including:

- Abdominal pain
- Diarrhea
- Intestinal bleeding
- Weight loss

Diagnostic tests for Crohn's include:

- Blood tests
- X-rays

If you're intent on obtaining a specifically named diagnosis, then it never hurts to have a colonoscopy. With all autoimmune conditions, however, the same positive agents and remedial protocols can be utilized to bring your body back into balance.

What causes Crohn's Disease?

While the cause of Crohn's disease remains uncertain, there's a substantial amount of evidence that genetic factors play an extremely important role in its development. The most widely accepted theory is that your immune system is overreacting to certain substances in your gut—most likely, to bacteria that are normally in the intestines—and that this overactive immune response is somehow triggering a reaction to something in your environment.

In other words, if you've developed Crohn's disease, then you have inherited some form of the defective gene or genes that cause your immune system to react in an abnormal way, leading to an influx of inflammatory cells into your intestine. There are a number of genes that can predispose you to develop the disease, and certain environmental factors can also affect its course.

While, unfortunately, the environmental factors have not been well studied, smoking and the use of nonsteroidal anti-inflammatory drugs (NSAIDs) have both been associated with the onset and severity of symptoms. Anything that alters the normal bacteria in your colon—even antibiotics or gastrointestinal infections—can put you at risk.

One of the most consistent risk factors for Crohn's disease is a diet high in refined sugar.

Sugar, which is derived from carbohydrates (fructose, sucrose, glucose) and milk (lactose) have a tendency to travel through the small intestine and colon and instead of getting passed out through the feces, in people with Crohn's, it has a tendency to travel through the remainder of the digestive tract and act as fuel for bacteria.

Several studies have shown that patients with Crohn's have increased amounts of carbohydrates in their diet.

Who gets Crohn's disease, and how common is it?

Recent estimates suggest that up to six hundred thousand people in the United States alone are affected by Crohn's disease. It appears to be more common in urban than in rural areas, and more in northern than southern areas. While Crohn's can occur at any age, it most commonly presents itself in people between the ages of twenty and thirty. As with ulcerative colitis, people of Jewish descent and from eastern European countries tend to be more affected than other populations.

Types of Crohn's Disease

The different types of Crohn's disease are based on its location in your body.

Gastroduodenal Crohn's Disease: Also known as upper GI Crohn's disease, this type is very uncommon, occurring in only about 5 percent of patients.

Jejunoileitis: Also uncommon, this type involves inflammation of the second part of the small intestine, the jejunum.

Ileitis: Occurring in about 30 percent of patients, this type involves inflammation of the last part of the small intestine, the ileum.

Ileocolitis: Affecting approximately 50 percent of Crohn's patients, this is the most common type of the disease. It involves inflammation of the ileum and the colon—most often the right side of the colon.

Crohn's Colitis: Approximately 20 percent of Crohn's patients suffer from this type, which involves inflammation of the colon only. Symptoms include diarrhea, rectal bleeding, and abdominal pain.

The MAP Gene

New evidence shows that a specific bacterium, *mycobacterium avium*, may be the causative agent in many cases of Crohn's disease. Mycobacterium avium subspecies *paratuberculosis*, which is from the same family as tuberculosis, is known as the MAP.

Robert J. Greenstein (2003) in *The Lancet* writes:

> *Although Crohn's disease is considered to be autoimmune in origin, there is increasing evidence that it may have an infectious cause . . . .*

> *The government of the UK has decided to exercise the precautionary principle concerning a possible link between Crohn's disease and MAP, and has decided to eradicate MAP from the food chain. This action is not contingent on demonstrating an unequivocal link between MAP and Crohn's disease . . . .*

> *MAP is found in the potable water supply of large cities in industrialised nations . . . .*

> *In animals, MAP causes Johne's disease, a chronic wasting intestinal diarrhoeal disease evocative of Crohn's disease. Johne's disease occurs in wild and domesticated animals, including dairy herds. Viable MAP is found in human and cow milk, and is not reliably killed by standard pasteurisation . . . .*

> *MAP in milk from domestic animals is well described, and it is not reproducibly eradicated by pasteurisation at the parameters*

routinely used in the USA. There are concerns that using pasteurisation standards effective against MAP may adversely affect the taste and, therefore, consumer acceptance of milk products. (507–508)

While the mere presence of a MAP DNA does not prove that MAP causes Crohn's disease, it's conceivable that when it is identified in human beings, the origin is pasteurized milk from cows that had Johne's disease.

According to a *PubMed* article on the National Center for Biotechnology Information (NCBI) website, while, "the evidence remains inconclusive . . . . Two main hypotheses exist with respect to the role of MAP in CD. The first is that MAP is a principal cause of CD, while the second is that MAP is more prevalent because of the immune dysfunction seen in CD but does not play a causative role" (Rosenfeld and Bressier, 2011).

We know that MAP is present, and we know that it can be a problem, yet we can't conclusively show that there's a causative link to Crohn's disease. Knowing that it could be a factor, however, and that other countries have used specific antibiotics to eradicate this mycobacterium, indicates that having it present in our bodies (depending on the level that is present) can cause serious problems.

Herding farmed animals together causes disease processes to be spread from one animal to another. When you ingest dairy and meat from infected animal sources (rather than grass-fed animals, organic stock, or free-range chickens) bacteria ultimately get passed on to you.

Once you become infected with a pathogen like the MAP gene, it can be very difficult to eliminate. Remember, 80 percent of your immune system is in your gut. You literally have trillions of different bacteria living in there. If only the proper bacteria are present, and all your body has to do is keep them in check, you'll be in a better position to decrease autoimmunity symptoms and improve your condition.

Why wait until you have a major infection?

Coffee Enemas

One unique way to help with digestive problems and to detoxify the colon and liver is via a coffee enema. Yes, you read that right.

Your liver deserves focused attention when you deal with autoimmune conditions. Toxicity that builds up in the liver can lead to increased inflammation.

Coffee enemas can help in many ways:

- Decrease inflammation
- Improve digestion
- Increase energy levels

The following is courtesy of Dr. Michael Johnson of Appleton, Wisconsin (2016):

> *While coffee is not ideal when digested the usual way there are some very beneficial herbal properties of coffee when taken rectally, and there are some overlap among these effects.*
>
> ***An astringent.*** *This is an herbal property that means it peels the top layer of skin or mucous membrane. This is helpful for some healing, as the top layer of skin or mucous membrane is often ready to come off anyway, and is loaded with toxins. So it is like cleaning the surface layer of the mucous membrane of the colon and the liver. Remember, your skin is the largest organ of your body, keep it healthy!*

A choleretic. *A choleretic is a substance that increases bile flow; which applies to coffee when used rectally. While other agents classed as choleretics increase bile flow from the liver, they do little to enhance detoxifying enzyme systems, and they do not ensure the passage of bile from the intestines out the rectum. Bile is normally reabsorbed up to nine or ten times before working its way out the intestines in feces. The enzyme enhancing ability of the coffee enema is unique among choleretics; because it does not allow as much reabsorption of toxic bile by the liver across the gut wall, it is a powerful means of detoxifying the blood stream through existing enzyme systems in the liver and small bowel. Clinical practice has shown coffee enemas to be well tolerated by patients when used as frequently as every four hours, the coffee enema may be classed as one of the only repeatable, non-reabsorbed, and effective choleretics in the medical literature.*

Enhancement of liver detoxification systems and glutathione production. *These are other general effects of coffee enemas that are explained in more detail below. Many times I will add glutathione from Premier Research Labs to the coffee for added benefit.*

Antioxidant effects. *Coffee contains powerful antioxidants. These are particularly helpful for the liver, which is highly subject to oxidant damage. Unlike common antioxidants such as vitamin C, alpha lipoic acid, selenium, zinc, vitamins A and E, the antioxidants in coffee are far more yang in Chinese medical terminology. This is a great advantage today because the bodies are already too yin and adding more yin antioxidants makes the problem much worse. Someday, doctors who recommend antioxidants will realize this problem with all antioxidant nutrients and will stop recommending so many of them, perhaps recommending the coffee enema instead.*

Reducing the need for antioxidants. Nutritional balancing and coffee retention enemas also reduce the need for antioxidants because they can remove the oxidant sources. This is far better than giving antioxidants. The oxidant sources are oxidized minerals including iron, copper, manganese and aluminum, among others.

Palmitic acids. In the late 1970s and early 1980s, researchers in the lab of Lee Wattenberg identified salts of palmitic acids (kahweol and cafestol palmitate) in coffee as potent enhancers of glutathione S-transferase, a major detoxification system that catalyzes the binding of a vast variety of electrophiles from the blood stream to the sulfhydryl group of glutathione. Because the reactive ultimate carcinogenic forms of chemicals are electrophiles, the glutathione S-transferase system must be regarded as an important mechanism for carcinogen detoxification.

By ensuring that you eat only good food, you can reduce your risk of exposure to pathogens that cause problems in your gut.

In addition to making better food choices, the most important things you can to do restore proper gut function are:

- Find, through the latest tests, the causes of any dysregulation in your intestinal system.

- Remove the causes of dysregulation through specific dietary changes.

- Repair the damaged tissues with specific nutritional supplements.

- Balance your immune system with specific nutrients and vitamins.

- Find, through neurological tests, imbalances in the frequency in firing of your brain.

- Improve your brain function with oxygen and brain-based therapy.

5

Rheumatoid Arthritis

CHARACTERISTICS AND DIAGNOSIS

Why is rheumatoid arthritis in an autoimmune book?

Isn't it just arthritis?

What is arthritis?

The word *arthro* means "joint", and *itis* means "inflammation". Arthritis is an inflammatory process around your joints, with two of the most common types being osteoarthritis (*osteo* meaning "bone") and rheumatoid arthritis. The difference between the two is that rheumatoid arthritis affects your blood as well.

Rheumatoid arthritis is a systemic problem because your immune system attacks the lining of the joints throughout your body, not just in one area. It's generally a painful disease.

Symptoms

Symptoms of rheumatoid arthritis include:

- Joint stiffness and swelling (swelling is caused by stiffness inhibiting your joints' range of motion)
- Reduced daily movement and function due to pain

- Fatigue
- Fever
- Weight loss
- Eye inflammation
- Lung disease
- Anemia

Rheumatoid arthritis is more common in women than in men, and it usually begins when you are over the age of forty.

How is it diagnosed?

Blood Testing and X-Rays

Diagnosing rheumatoid arthritis does not just involve an exam; it requires a good clinical history, a good clinical examination, and additional testing, including blood tests. We run a *citrullinated peptide antibody* test to look for a rheumatoid factor (RF) in the blood. If the rheumatoid factor is present, then we know that you have rheumatoid arthritis. When you're aging and you have the symptoms of arthritis, you might assume that you have rheumatoid arthritis. But unless that RF is present in your blood, it's osteoarthritis.

Other things we look for in your bloodwork include the erythrocyte sedimentation rate (ESR), C-reactive protein, and your white blood cell count.

X-rays are another diagnostic tool that we use to determine exactly what kind of arthritic condition you have. Unfortunately, some of the signs, such as joint damage, generally occur in the later stages of the disease, and by the time you present with these symptoms, the problems have already set in.

Other Indicators

As mentioned previously, the function of your adrenal glands (your stress glands located above your kidneys) is extremely important. When there's a problem with your adrenals, the release of cortisol and DHEA is compromised. This can cause an increase in intestinal permeability, which could lead to leaky gut syndrome (see the chapter on gastrointestinal issues) and could be an indicator of rheumatoid arthritis or another form of autoimmune disease.

Other indicators could include:

- Fatty acid imbalance
- Oxidative stress
- Hormone imbalances

Because this is a systemic illness, it affects your whole body.

RISKS AND COMPLICATIONS

According to Johns Hopkins Arthritis Center, 1 to 2 percent of the world's population is affected by rheumatoid arthritis, its prevalence increases with age, and forty-one out of every hundred thousand people in the United States are diagnosed with RA. The diagnosis is more common than multiple sclerosis or even leukemia.

There are a number of factors that can predispose you to having rheumatoid arthritis.

Smoking: Rheumatoid arthritis is four times more common in smokers than in non-smokers, with smoking being a major contributor to oxidative stress on your body.

Periodontal Disease: Periodontal (gum) disease, a chronic oral infection caused by inflammatory reactions to certain bacteria, affects approximately 35 to 50 percent of adults and can increase the incidence of rheumatoid arthritis. Treating any incidences of periodontal disease can therefore improve your rheumatoid arthritis outcomes.

Acidity: Your body's pH level is extremely important. Low pH means low oxygen levels throughout your body. (Remember that your total body pH is different from your blood pH, which doesn't change much.) Your total body pH should be somewhere between 6.4 and 7.0. If it goes below 6.4, your body becomes more acidic, and an acidic environment is a breeding ground for problems, including those associated with rheumatoid arthritis.

Joint Deformation: Over time, the increased frequency of rheumatoid arthritis flare-ups leads to joint deformation. Your joints can actually shift out of place, which can be very painful.

Osteoporosis: Rheumatoid arthritis and the medications associated with its treatment can weaken your bones and lead to the possibility of osteoporosis.

Carpal Tunnel Syndrome: With rheumatoid arthritis, we see an increase in the incidence of carpal tunnel syndrome. The carpal tunnel runs between the two rows of bone in your wrist. If there is rheumatoid arthritis and the bones shift a little bit, that can compromise the tunnel and cause numbness or tingling in the fingers and hands or, in some cases, a lot of pain.

Heart Problems and Lung Disease: Other complications associated with rheumatoid arthritis include heart problems and lung disease. Many people experience scarring of lung tissue. A report in the *Journal of Arthritis Research and Therapy* states that rheumatoid arthritis sufferers are at an increased risk of death if they also suffer from coronary artery disease. According to Dr. Mark Gostine, founder of Michigan Pain Consultants, inflammation of the arteries allows increased space for buildup of plaque leading to artery disease and highly increased risk of heart disease. If you are suffering from rheumatoid arthritis, you are at risk for heart disease problems as well.

Environmental Triggers and Gut Flora: According to a 2008 *Journal of Rheumatology* editorial by Dr. Christopher J. Edwards, an MD, Consultant Rheumatologist, and Honorary Senior Lecturer in the Department of Rheumatology at Southampton University Hospitals NHS Trust in the United Kingdom:

> *The important environmental drivers of RA are still being sought. However, it is conceivable that different compositions of gut flora may alter the normal physiological interactions within the intestine and expose the immune system to bacterial antigens with arthritogenic potential. Perhaps when looking for microbial triggers for RA in the environment we need to spend time looking at our most common exposure to bacteria in the form of the abundant commensal bacteria teeming on and in us every day.*

How might changes in gut flora produce changes in the immune system or immune function that may lead to inflammatory joint disease?

Studies show that problems with gut flora can potentially lead to rheumatoid arthritis. As with all autoimmune conditions, your gut is extremely important because that's where 80 percent of your immune system is.

When immunologist Dr. Dan Littman of New York University tested fecal samples from New York City residents, he found that a bacterium called *Prevotella copri* was present in the intestines of 75 percent of the patients who had been diagnosed with rheumatoid arthritis but hadn't yet been treated for it (Scher et al., 2013).

Do you think this might explain the reported improvement of rheumatoid arthritis symptoms in individuals who started on a vegetarian, gluten-free, or dairy-free diet?

Could their symptoms be improving because they are clearing out their guts?

TREATMENTS

What are some of the treatments for people suffering from rheumatoid arthritis?

Currently, the standard medical approach to treating rheumatoid arthritis is the pharmaceutical dispensing of medications in an attempt to decrease inflammation, such as:

- Methotrexate
- Sulfasalazine
- Azathioprine
- Penicillamine
- Corticosteroids
- COX-2 inhibitors

But this is only a temporary solution. It does not correct the problem.

You may have seen television commercials for products like Enbrel (etanercept). These types of drugs are just a quick fix with side effects. They won't correct your rheumatoid arthritis. They might decrease the flare-ups or temporarily decrease some of the pain, but that does not correct the problem.

When you have an autoimmune condition or any kind of abnormal physiological response, there are always free radicals involved. Free radical production causes problems like cancer.

What can you do about that?

Glutathione Supplementation

To decrease inflammation, we recommend you use supplements such as a glutathione. Glutathione is the number-one antioxidant in your body. It reduces the free radical damage from any autoimmune condition.

We also recommend:

- Calcium
- Zinc
- Magnesium
- Selenium

These are all important in the treatment of rheumatoid arthritis.

Other products that may be helpful include:

- Resveratrol
- Curcumin
- Green tea extract

Increased inflammation causes increased pain. In order to decrease the pain associated with rheumatoid arthritis, we need to decrease the inflammatory response. The following supplements can help with reducing inflammation.

EPA and DHA: Essential fatty acids like eicosapentaenoic acid (EPA) and docosahexaenoic acid (DHA) are extremely important in the daily treatment of rheumatoid arthritis. They're found in fish oils and krill oil.

Vitamin D3: While it's always best to get the nutrients you need straight from the source of your natural environment, the vitamin D that you need to stay healthy comes from the sun, and most of us don't get enough sun exposure. For example, if you're staying inside during cold winters, you need to supplement with vitamin D. Vitamin D3 is extremely beneficial in the treatment of rheumatoid arthritis. For more on vitamin D3, see the "Treatments" section in the next chapter.

CoCurcumin: CoCurcumin is a combination of coenzyme Q10 (CoQ10) and curcumin, a natural anti-inflammatory derived from turmeric. The great thing about CoCurcumin is that it's not just targeted toward one specific joint or for short-term relief like Advil or Naproxen, but it works on the inflammatory process globally, throughout your entire body.

Because rheumatoid arthritis is a systemic problem, it's important to take a systemic approach to treatment. Generally, the disease is treated symptomatically because people don't know there's a problem until they experience pain. By the time you have pain, the inflammatory process has already set in. By taking a systemic approach, you can prevent inflammation from happening and get much better results.

6

Multiple Sclerosis

PROBLEMS, CAUSES, AND TRIGGERS

Multiple sclerosis (MS) is another autoimmune disease that can be extremely debilitating. With MS, your body's immune system starts to destroy the outer layer of your nerves, called the *myelin sheath*.

Myelin is a fatty substance that helps your nerves to send information to one another and to and from the brain. Its presence is necessary for all communication that occurs throughout your entire body. When *demyelination* (a loss of the myelin sheath) occurs, your nerves' frequency of firing (FOF) decreases, and when this happens, too much stimulation in the form of hot or cold can cause an increase in your symptoms. Due to the demyelination process there can be a buildup of plaque or lesions containing inflammatory cells.

The *lesions*, or scar tissue from nerve damage, of MS typically originate in the optic nerve. They also come from the spinal cord, the brainstem, and the *white matter* (myelin and nerve fibers) of the cerebral hemispheres in your brain. When MS is present and your nerves have a decreased FOF, your body cannot allow the tissues to heal or the nerves to fire properly.

Metabolic Capacity

When there's too much stimulation, your body can exceed its *metabolic capacity*, or the amount of stimuli it can process without experiencing any adverse effects (referred to as EMC for *exceeded metabolic capacity*). Once you reach or exceed that metabolic capacity, your nervous system can't handle any more stimuli. At that point, there is nothing else you can do for the day, just rest.

Because people with MS typically have a very low metabolic capacity, the increased heart rate or sweating from too much stimulation or exercise can cause problems. If you have MS, you should avoid excessive exercise.

What causes MS?

The causes of MS can be:

- Environmental
- Hereditary
- Linked to issues with the metabolic process

Reactions to certain types of foods or products may be precursors to MS. While research has not yet shown this definitively, based on the outcomes of clinical studies, it is believed that the following substances could contribute to the onset of multiple sclerosis.

Aspartame

Aspartame is an extremely toxic substance found in products like NutraSweet, Equal, Spoonful, and a multitude of diet soft drinks.

Although aspartame is used in many diet-related products, it does not cause you to lose weight. It can actually cause you to gain weight by turning off your body's satiety centers — the centers in your brain that tell your body when you're full. As aspartame tricks your body into thinking that you're not full, you start to crave carbohydrates, and as you eat more carbohydrates, you gain more weight.

Consumption of aspartame can cause seizures and can also cause changes in your body's dopamine levels. This can be deadly if you suffer from Parkinson's disease.

How does this relate to MS?

As mentioned in the chapter on diabetes, at higher temperatures, aspartame — or its derivative, wood alcohol — is converted to formaldehyde. Formaldehyde is a preservation agent; it's used to preserve cadavers for dissection in medical school anatomy labs. When aspartame is converted to formaldehyde in your body, the formaldehyde is then converted to formic acid, which leads to metabolic acidosis. This may be a precursor to two types of autoimmune disease: *systemic lupus erythematosus* (more commonly known as lupus) and multiple sclerosis.

It is possible that some people may have symptoms similar to MS when they actually have too much aspartame or they develop aspartame toxicity. Once this issue is resolved then the symptoms that look like MS may disappear. But the fact that long-term toxic exposure may progress to something more substantial such as MS is still a possibility.

Oral Contraceptives

Other possible causes of multiple sclerosis are oral contraceptives.

According to a Fox News health article:

> *In a new study, researchers found an increased risk of multiple sclerosis (MS) among women who have taken oral contraceptives . . . .*

> *Utilizing membership data from Kaiser Permanente Southern California, researchers analyzed the health records of 305 women aged 14 to 48 who were diagnosed with MS or its precursor, clinically isolated syndrome (CIS), between 2008 and 2011. They looked at the women's birth control use up to three years prior to the onset of MS symptoms.*

> *Overall, researchers found a 30 percent increased risk of developing MS amongst women who had at least three months of oral contraceptive use, compared to a control group of 3,050 women who did not have MS.* (Kwan, 2014)

This does not mean that oral contraceptives are a cause of MS, but it does indicate a direct link.

Processed Table Salt

Processed salt is a horrible thing. I've mentioned sugar being called *white death*, and I consider salt to be just as bad. White processed sugar and salt can't be metabolized properly without side effects. Processed table salt and even the sea salt that you see in stores (not to be confused with *aleae*, a pink sea salt from Hawaii) have been shown to lead to an increase in multiple sclerosis and other autoimmune-related diseases.

Markus Kleinewietfeld, PhD, Department of Neurology and Immunology at the Yale School of Medicine, led a study that showed that a higher physiological state of salt (NaCl) *in vivo* markedly boosted the induction of interleukin (IL-17), producing CD4+ helper T cells that have been associated with autoimmune disease. The study also suggests that adding salt to the diet of mice induced Th17 cells (a type of helper T cells), and that mice with a high-salt diet developed a more severe form of the animal model of MS (Kleinewietfeld et al., 2013).

Bacterial Toxins

Bacterial toxins may also trigger MS. One is called *clostridium perfringens Type B*, which carries a gene that can produce what are known as *epsilon toxins*. Researchers from the Weill Cornell Medical College identified the toxin in a twenty-one-year-old woman who had flare-ups of MS (Weill Cornell, 2013).

Although not unusual in certain animals, for this specific bacterium to be found in a human being is highly significant, according to researchers. Clostridium perfringens Type A is quite common, but Type B is found in soil and in the intestinal tracts of grass-eating animals, not normally in humans. These bacteria sit in the animal's gut and make the *epsilon toxin*, causing problems. One reason we don't typically see epsilon toxins in humans is because the intestinal tracts of the animals are a different shape from humans'. In humans, clostridium perfringens Type B does not grow well because we have what's called a *linear tract*, or a straight line.

When researchers detected the toxin in the woman mentioned above, they hypothesized there may be a connection to MS because damage from the toxin in animals targets the same tissues as those damaged by MS.

Geography

The Mayo Clinic did a study that shows if a child moves from a high-risk area to a low-risk area or vice versa, the child actually tends to acquire the risk level associated with the new home area. But if the move occurs after puberty, the young adult retains the risk level associated with his or her first home.

SYMPTOMS AND TESTING

If you have multiple sclerosis, you may experience associated symptoms, such as double vision, blurred vision, or loss of vision (usually in one eye), and numbness or tingling anywhere in the body. Another symptom generally occurs if you tilt your chin toward your chest, bending your neck forward. If a shock-like feeling occurs at that time, that may be indicative of multiple sclerosis.

Other symptoms of MS include:

- Uncontrollable tremors or movement disorders
- Balance problems
- Difficulty walking
- Slurred speech
- Fatigue
- Dizziness
- Heat sensitivity

How are we able to determine if your suffering is actually from multiple sclerosis?

As we see from the list of common symptoms, MS can be very similar to a lot of other problems. Consult your health care practitioner who can determine if you do fall within a clinical diagnosis of multiple sclerosis. To make a clear diagnosis will require a battery of different tests and clinical workups by various specialists.

Neurologic Examination

A neurological examination is a key screening tool for diagnosis of MS. The neurologist—whether a chiropractic neurologist or a medical neurologist—will check your optic nerves by looking in your eyes for a condition called optic neuritis. That is the first area affected by multiple sclerosis.

The practitioner should complete a comprehensive neurological examination, looking at reflexes and checking for *Lhermitte's sign*, the sensation of electrical shock at the forward bending of the neck I described earlier. This is generally the first indication that multiple sclerosis may be the appropriate diagnosis.

Bloodwork

Examining the blood for autoimmune response correlates the diagnosis with other findings.

Spinal Tap

Doctors may perform a spinal tap to look for abnormalities within the spinal fluid. They want to rule out viral infection in the spinal cord and throughout the nervous system.

Magnetic Resonance Imaging (MRI)

MRI stands for *Magnetic Resonance Imaging*. The region of your body that needs to be viewed is placed within a large, magnetic imaging tube. The huge magnet causes slight movement in the hydrogen atoms of the area of your body inside the tube. These movements are picked up by radio waves that are received and integrated into an actual image of the soft tissues in your body. The appropriate practitioner views these images and can diagnose any abnormalities, not just in the bones as with an

X-ray, but more important, within soft tissues such as those found in the brain and spinal cord.

The radiologist can see any pathological lesions. When these pathologies are seen in the spinal cord and there is evidence of plaquing (loss of the protective myelin sheath), this is generally indicative of a multiple sclerosis diagnosis.

A proper diagnosis for MS cannot be made after just one test.

It requires a multitude of avenues of tests and factors, combining:

- History
- Examination
- Diagnostic imaging
- Bloodwork

All have to be factored into the mix in order to make a proper diagnosis.

RISK FACTORS AND COMPLICATIONS

There are certain risk factors associated with, or precursors to, multiple sclerosis:

- **Age:** The risk of developing multiple sclerosis is greatest between the ages of twenty and forty.

- **Sex**: Multiple sclerosis occurs more frequently in women than men.

- **Family History:** If anybody in your family has an autoimmune condition — and that holds true with all autoimmune conditions — then that makes you more likely to have or inherit any other kind of autoimmune condition. If you have any autoimmune condition described in this book, then you may be potentially at risk for any of the other autoimmune conditions listed here.

- **Viral Infections:** If you suffer from something like Epstein-Barr virus, you are at greater risk for multiple sclerosis as well.

- **Ethnicity:** The predominance of multiple sclerosis occurs generally in Caucasians, specifically of northern European heritage. There's an increased incidence in areas such as Canada and Northern Europe. It is much less prevalent in South America, Central America, and Asia. We also see a prevalence of it in New Zealand. It occurs farther from the equator and closer to the poles, not so much in warmer climates.

Flare-Ups

It is usual to experience ups and downs, relapses, and remissions with multiple sclerosis. Generally, extreme heat is going to cause flare-ups. This is why if you have MS, we don't want you exercising excessively. We want to make sure that you are generally as comfortable as possible throughout the progression of this disease. MS does not have a cure, but we can make sure that we mediate it as much as possible. We can try to control the symptoms as well as some of the causes in order to make sure that you live a full, healthy life.

Further complications can include:

- Paralysis
- Issues affecting bladder and bowel function
- Issues affecting sexual organs and sexual response
- Muscle stiffness and spasms
- Depression
- Epilepsy

TREATMENTS

Treatments in the medical community for multiple sclerosis are mostly focused on the administration of corticosteroids and immunosuppressants. This is generally the same as treatments for autoimmune conditions from the medical community.

When an autoimmune condition is present, the medical community's strategy is often to suppress the immune system even more. This seems to be the limit of what they have in their toolbox. They may not be aware of other treatments or other protocols that exist in order to help with autoimmune-related conditions. Therefore, what they are doing isn't really *wrong*, but they most likely do not understand what other options are available.

Alternative or Functional Neurologic Therapies

Alternative or functional neurology employs many therapies that target the creation and strengthening of new neural pathways. Movement is a very effective therapy. For example, a *wobble board* is a simple piece of equipment that is a flat, plywood disc attached to a curved bottom. The curved bottom causes the board to wobble when you stand on it. You have to balance using gross-motor movements. This kind of activity stimulates specific regions in the brain and causes neurological growth and change, helping the areas affected by MS. Movement is also combined with other therapies for greater effect.

Cryotherapy

Ice therapy or *cryotherapy* is the act of applying cold in order to decrease pain and inflammation. Currently there are new studies underway with regards to whole-body cryotherapy. This may be something that could change in the future. In general, I'm not an advocate of the ice therapy that many doctors recommend because ice therapy doesn't just stop the pain; it stops the nerves from firing. By slowing down the FOF, it stops the healing process.

Metronome Therapy

We can target specific regions in the brain by guiding you to coordinate your movements with an *interactive metranome*. The metranome audibly clicks regular beats, anywhere from forty to sixty beats per minute. Using the metranome as the guide, you do a specific movement, such as touching a dot on the wall and then your nose, or bouncing a ball, or other patterned movements. Doing this in time with the metronome increases the frequency of firing of the neurons in the affected area of the brain.

Eye Pursuits and Eye Movements

As mentioned earlier, problems with vision are a common occurrence with multiple sclerosis. *Optic neuritis* is inflammation of the optic nerve. We want to make sure to stimulate and increase the firing of nerves affected by this condition. Your doctor may suggest exercising your eyes with *pursuits*, in which you follow the doctor's finger or your own finger through a series of specific movements or other eye exercises such as *saccades* (rapid eye movement between fixed points) and *antisaccades*.

Exercise with Oxygen Therapy

The brain needs two things to survive: it needs fuel and activation. Fuel comes in the form of glucose and oxygen. Exercise is good medicine and it is made even better with supplemental oxygen.

Why do we need to add oxygen?

Your ability to utilize oxygen declines markedly—by about 1 percent every year—after age twenty-five. We want to make sure that you're getting enough oxygen as you exercise.

To boost the amount of oxygen available, we use an oxygen concentrator. An oxygen concentrator takes approximately 90 percent of the oxygen out of the air and concentrates it through a filter; this comes in through a cannula. When you put the cannula on, you receive oxygen at a rate of three to five liters per minute. I've successfully treated many patients with this therapy.

You can do any kind of exercise. In my practice I have an upper body ergometer, described in the fibromyalgia chapter. The upper body ergometer is a fitness machine that requires you to crank two opposing handles, much in the same way you might use your feet to pedal a bicycle. It is efficient both in terms of time and space and gives the user an appropriate amount of activity.

Why work the upper body?

The closer we get to your brain, the more receptors there are, and the greater potential for healing.

By doing this movement, in which your arms are moving in opposition, you are actually stimulating the spinal-cerebellar pathways. These are powerful pathways that send information to the brain from your upper body.

You should do this exercise for anywhere from five to ten minutes. Remember, you don't want to create a high-stress movement that will induce sweat or cause you to feel excessively hot. This is not an aerobic movement, meaning that all you're doing is firing all the right centers, not getting a workout from this.

Vibration

Vibration is a very powerful tool when applied to the cerebellum. Vibration will stimulate the dorsal columns of the spinal cord. Specifically when a stimulus such as vibration is applied, it stimulates an ascending pathway or spinal tract going to the brain. This pathway goes through the dorsal column medial lemniscus and sends information up to the thalamus and finally to the post central gyrus and somatosensory cortex of the brain.

Vitamin D3

In 2013, Jean Bardot of the online *Natural News* reported then-recent findings regarding vitamin D3 and sunlight: "The *Journal of Neurology, Neurosurgery, and Psychiatry* with *Practical Neurology* explains that supplementation with Vitamin D3 and exposure to the sun may reduce the risk of developing multiple sclerosis."

Vitamin D3 and calcium are related throughout many different body functions and they work together. D3 can help to promote intestinal calcium as well as aiding in the cardiovascular function. It may also help maintain the health of the cell and healthy cell metabolism. If you experience a drop in D3, your body will be unable to metabolize calcium properly. The study further suggests that vitamin D3 is very helpful in slowing the degenerative process of MS and can help in prevention of MS.

In conclusion, diet and nutrition are extremely important and valuable in the treatment of patients suffering from multiple sclerosis. Activation of the nervous system is also essential. Simply taking immunosuppressants to decrease the frequency of neuronal firing in associated deficient areas of the brain is not going to be the best thing for you. You do not want to exceed metabolic capacity. You want to be able to treat all areas affected accordingly.

Multiple Sclerosis Case: Dr. Robert McCarthy, DC (Greenville, North Carolina)

Email received from patient with MS:

Greetings from Italy!

We are moving deeper into the program and only have two weeks to go so I thought I would dash off a few lines and give you an update. Kelly has gone back to meet some responsibilities at ECU. I have put in some long days and continue to pace myself as best I can — sometimes pushing a bit too hard not wanting to miss anything.

I am pleased to report that in March during the spring break I climbed to the top of Mount Vesuvius! I did this in high wind and cold temperatures after being on my feet all morning with a two-and-a-half-hour tour of Pompeii. Felt like a good personal accomplishment and a recognition that I have come a long way. When the MS first hit, I could only stand up for about fifteen minutes at a time.

I am discovering that gluten free in Italy sometimes means that they switch from wheat to a corn flower — in my case just as bad. So I am trying to fine-tune what I am putting into me but suspect that there are some subtle ways I might be polluting myself and need to be on top of it at all times. Restaurants have been very helpful about offering alternatives — last night a fine soup followed by a dish of white beans and celery with some onions and olive oil. When I am on the move I am usually quite content with grilled vegetables, salads, and chicken, etc.

Thank you again for all your help in getting me to this point — if I had not put in the time and work and gotten myself to a point that I felt reasonably comfortable, I doubt if I would have taken on this trip.

7

Healing Autoimmunity

Your body's state of being or *homeostasis* responds to many types of stimuli. When these stimuli impact your body's various systems, they are known as *stressors*. There are many different stressors, both negative and positive, and they all have an impact on your health.

If and when we see stressors that have a negative impact on the body, we can localize and target the affected areas. Then we can come up with an effective treatment protocol based on where in the nervous system and metabolic system there may be compromises. We must therefore create an environment that is beneficial to our health and well-being and in turn negate certain stressors, such as harmful bacteria strains and immune-modifying factors that can directly or indirectly impact immunity.

METHYLATION

Methylation, also mentioned in the fibromyalgia chapter, is an essential chemical process that occurs in your body on a cellular level. Its optimal or less-than-optimal functioning affects regulatory processes.

All autoimmune conditions are impacted by methylation. Therefore, it's important for you to know how to support healthy function.

Methylation is very important for the following processes:

- DNA/RNA synthesis (i.e., turning on/off genes)
- Neurotransmitter production (e.g., dopamine and serotonin)
- Hormonal breakdown (e.g., estrogen and testosterone)
- Creation of immune cells (e.g., NK cells and T-cells)
- Creation of protective coating on nerves (i.e., myelin formation)
- Processing chemicals and toxins (detoxification)

How do you know whether you should be concerned about methylation in your body?

Here's a list of symptoms, divided into categories.

Category 1:

- Fatigue
- Slow Recovery from exercise
- Slow healing following injury
- Difficulty with weight loss
- Slow metabolism
- Low muscle tone

Category 2:

- Focus/concentration issues
- Mood instability
- Sleep disturbances (waking up often)
- Clumsiness
- Loss of train of thought
- Mixing up words when speaking or writing

- Trouble with organizational skills
- History of ADD/ADHD

Category 3:

- Chronic infections
- Yeast overgrowth
- History of bacterial or fungal infections
- Gut issues (bowel irritation, constipation, diarrhea)
- Chronic sinus infections
- Need for multiple doses of antibiotics

The category your symptoms are found in can give you a clue for which direction to take when trying to heal.

Left untreated or unsupported, poor methylation can have big consequences, including:

- Cancer

- Neurological disorders such as anxiety, depression, Parkinson's, tremor disorder, MS, Alzheimer's, dementia, neuropathies, migraines, and cluster headaches

- Hormonal regulation issues such as PMS, ovarian cysts, fibroids, Polycystic Ovary Syndrome (PCOS) in women or low testosterone in men

- Chemical sensitivities

- Autoimmune disorders and immune deficiencies such as fibromyalgia, chronic fatigue syndrome, ADHD, autism, Asperger's syndrome, dyslexia, and learning differences

- Insomnia

Methylation Protocols

The following list is intended to provide general information about products available from several different suppliers. Please consult a health professional before using any of these products. Do not attempt to diagnose and prescribe on your own.

Neuro-Immune Stabilizer: (cream) This supplement is applied first with a loading dose, then tapers off after that. You may notice the red color of the cream. It's red because of the methylated B vitamins.

In addition to the Neuro-Immune Stabilizer, the following products may help, depending on your symptoms.

Mitochondrial Restore: (capsules) if you have two or more symptoms from Category 1.

Advanced Neurotransmitter Support: (capsules) can help if you have two or more symptoms from Category 2. The best time to take this product is in the morning with food.

Neuro-Immune Infection Control: (capsules) if you have two or more symptoms from Category 3.

Methyl Folate Plus: (capsules) these are used to address the problem of folate receptor antibodies, MTHFR polymorphism, increased tetrahydrofolate development, recovery from a major neurological injury, an inability to tolerate topical applications of these ingredients, and moderate to severe neuro-immune syndromes.

Glutathione Plus: (cream) used for chronic fatigue, high cholesterol, chemotherapy toxicity, autism spectrum disorders, heavy metal toxicity.

Calming Cream: used for relaxation, nervousness, sleep disturbances, difficulty falling asleep.

THERAPIES

Many patients who suffer from chronic neurologic conditions have areas of decreased cortical or cerebellar function. Imbalances in brain function indicate areas of decreased cellular health in the brain. As neurons in the brain degenerate, the body's ability to function may become impaired. When there is an area of the brain that fails to function as efficiently as it should, other areas of the brain begin to overfire. It causes imbalance and dysfunction in the body. Brain-based therapies are used to rehabilitate the specific area of decreased function. Following are some of the therapies that I typically offer patients in my practice.

Adjustments and Manipulation:

Coupled Reduction Unilateral Adjustments: These are bio-mechanically correct, hands-on adjustments. This technique is safe and is the most stimulation your brain can receive from a single treatment. Adjusting the extremities offers the least brain stimulation while adjusting the neck offers the most. We treat unilaterally because we want to focus on the side of the brain that is deficient in its firing.

Activator Adjustments: The activator is a small, handheld, spring-loaded instrument that allows me to give impulse-type adjustments to the joints and surrounding musculature. The repetitive impulses create multiple stretch reflexes in the muscles around your spine that fire into the brain. This is a more gentle approach and extremely safe for children and the elderly.

Vibration Therapy: This instrument saturates the tissues with a combination of vibration and percussion. It feels great, and helps to increase blood and lymph flow in the tissues. It also helps to break up adhesions left in the muscles from old chronic injuries. Vibration sensation is carried through the dorsal spino-cerebellar pathways and stimulates the cerebellum on the same side to which it is applied. This is an extremely powerful tool to stimulate the cerebellum and the rest of the brain.

Brain-Based Therapies

Posture-Pump Traction Therapy: The posture pump works by supporting the cervical curve while you perform extension exercises against light resistance. The posture pump inflates under your neck and will re-train your cerebellum to restore the normal lordotic curve in the neck.

Wobble Chair: Sit on this chair with your feet flat on the floor. Try to keep your chest and upper torso steady while you move your hips and pelvis in a figure-eight pattern. Then reverse the figure-eights. Spend three minutes each visit performing your wobble chair exercises.

Peripheral Neuropathy Rehabilitation Therapy (PNRT), a.k.a. Rebuilder Therapy: Just as with diabetes and fibromyalgia, PNRT is an effective form of therapy for many other autoimmune conditions. It provides nerve-based electrical stimulation that runs at 7.83 hertz and is designed to rehabilitate damaged nerve tissue. It stimulates large-diameter afferent nerves, thereby decreasing pain and increasing the ability to feel the extremities (hands, feet) and regain sensation. It may decrease numbness and tingling associated with different forms of neuropathy.

Metronome Therapy: This therapy, also mentioned in the previous chapter, works on the body and mind simultaneously in a motivating and engaging way while addressing critical timing skills that underlie all of our human capabilities:

- Speech
- Language
- Attention
- Memory
- Learning
- Reading
- Motor skills
- Self-control

As timing in the brain becomes more synchronous through metronome training, the brain's efficiency and performance also improves.

This leads to gains in many areas:

- Focus
- Cognitive speed
- Language processing
- Reading achievement
- Motor skills such as coordination, gait, and balance

BrainPaint Neurofeedback: Neurofeedback (also called *neurotherapy*) is a non-invasive process in which brain waves are monitored in real time by a computer, which can then use that information to produce changes in brainwave activity. The process of adjusting brainwave activity is known as *operant conditioning*, a method in which rewards for positive behavior increase learning capabilities. Read more about this revolutionary treatment at my website: www.neurologix.ca or www.brainpaint.com.

Electrical Muscle Stimulation: This therapy is used to reduce muscle spasms. It produces endorphins and enkephalins, which are natural pain relievers within your body.

Neuromuscular Re-education: This describes procedures used to retrain dysfunctional muscles throughout your body. It aids in the stabilization of joints that are weak and dysfunctional.

We use several pieces of equipment in this training:

- Wobble Board
- Balance Beam
- Trampoline

We also guide you to learn and use what are called *complex non-linear movements*. These are movements of limbs in the form of a figure-eight or modified version of that type of movement. This movement is beneficial in stimulating the contra-lateral or opposite brain, specifically the parietal lobe. This lobe of the brain's function deals with somato-sensory information.

Eyelight Therapy: This light-based therapy targets and rehabilitates areas of cortical degeneration in the brain.

Oxygen Therapy: Oxygen Concentrators, as described in the previous chapter, supply oxygen-enriched air in order to support proper brain function. We typically use a five-milliliter flow rate. This is approximately 90 percent oxygen. It is extremely safe.

Caloric Therapy: Using cold or hot water in your ear stimulates the vestibular system and the cerebellum. This can be an effective treatment if you have balance disorders and severe chronic pain.

Upper Body Ergometer (UBE): This machine is gives your upper body a workout, much in the same way that a bicycle works your legs; you pedal with your arms. As described in the fibromyalgia chapter, this stimulates the cuneocerebellar tract. It is more powerful because it stimulates more receptors that are closer in proximity to the brain than the spinocerebellar tract (for the legs). The closer we are to the brain, the more receptors that we fire.

Pursuit Exercises: These are slow tracking exercises for the eyes. You follow a moving target with your gaze and this stimulates the brain.

Optokinetic Tape: The use of this red and white tape or iPad program has two functions: diagnostic and therapeutic. First, it helps to identify through movement of the eyes what part of the brain is not functioning properly. Second, it helps correct the affected area. The parietal lobe moves the eyes to the same side, the frontal lobe refixates the eyes back, and the cerebellum stops them from moving.

Spin Therapy with Fixation: When you spin to the right in a chair, you stimulate the right cerebellum. If you fix your eyes on an object, you will be more able to do the movement without getting dizzy.

HEALING WITH SUPPLEMENTS AND NUTRICEUTICALS

The goal in dealing with diet and supplementation is to allow you to experience overall better health. This can happen within the organization of your organs by improving their physiological function. Whenever dealing with chronic inflammatory conditions, such as in autoimmune diseases, it is imperative that you remove the major triggers of inflammation in the body. There are certain foods and supplements that contribute to this anti-inflammatory process in a significant way. Nutraceuticals are supplements derived usually from plant and food sources. Like pharmaceuticals, they provide medicinal benefit, but without the synthetics and chemicals produced in a lab.

Taurine: This amino acid is the most abundant amino acid in the brain, heart, and nervous system. It is vital in helping the body to detoxify chemicals that may be harmful. It is also extremely important in helping the liver to function at its highest capacity.

Glutathione: It is the number one antioxidant in your body. Glutathione is vital in protecting your body against damage from free radicals, the precursors to cancer. It is extremely helpful in the daily function of the liver. One of the best ways to deliver glutathione is through the feet. When you use a cream like Oxicell from Apex Industries, you get the maximum benefits of glutathione. We can also try to promote our natural production of glutathione with products such as Glutathione Recycler (also from Apex). Glutathione Plus from Neurobiologix is another wonderful product that has great results.

Garlic: Allicin is the compound found in garlic that gives it all of its health benefits.

CoQ10: Coenzyme Q10 is vital in combating antioxidants. Ubiquinol is the active form. The use of CoQ10 is essential for proper heart health.

Betaine Hcl: Derived from beets, this dietary supplement helps with the regulation of pH in the stomach. By having adequate stomach acid, this allows the body to break down food and utilize vitamins such as B12 and minerals such as calcium, iron, and many others.

Curcumin: Curcumin is derived from turmeric. This supplement helps to support a healthy liver, colon, all cells, heart, and musculoskeletal system. It is a natural anti-inflammatory and a key product in the treatment of all of my patients. In my clinic I use CoCurcumin from Ayush Herbs. I find that their combination of CoQ10 and Curcumin to be the most effective natural anti-inflammatory at this time.

Resveratrol: Resveratrol is an immune booster and anti-inflammatory. It deeply penetrates the center of the cells' nucleii, giving DNA time to repair free radical damage. It's the resveratrol that's present in red wine and dark chocolate that makes people say ingesting them is beneficial—but taking them in the more potent form of a supplement is much simpler.

Resveratrol acts in many ways:

- Antioxidant
- Gastrointestinal support
- Detoxification
- Liver support
- Blood metabolism support
- Immune system modulation
- Balanced support for the body's natural inflammatory response

Chaga: Chaga is a form of mushroom. Research on Chaga has reported potent anti-viral properties. Two studies on its use on influenza virus and HIV were published with positive results in 1996. Chaga is thought to work on viruses indirectly by enhancing the human immune system as indicated by two papers published in 2002 and 2005. Historical use of Chaga as an anti-inflammatory may be attributed to that same mechanism. An alcohol extraction of Chaga was reported to lower elevated blood sugar levels. Chaga also contains powerful antioxidants.

Robin's Chaga makes alcohol extract with the Chaga mushroom. See www.robinschaga.com.

Nitric Balance: As a diabetic, I find this product to be vital on a daily basis. This trademarked product from Apex Industries was developed to provide the key nutrients for the expression and balance of the Inducible Nitric Oxide Synthase (iNOS) system. iNOS is key in cellular destruction. It does have some benefits though, such as increasing Endothelial Nitric Oxide Synthase (eNOS) and Neurogenic Nitric Oxide Synthase (nNos).

The primary role of eNOS is to aid in relaxing blood vessels. It is an anti-inflammatory and will also dilate the blood vessels to maximize blood flow to the extremities and sexual organs. This is great for exercise, rehabilitation, and overall health of the cardiovascular system.

Xanthinol Nicotinate: This is a vasodilator, therefore it will increase the amount of blood flowing to an area.

N-Acetyl L-Carnitine: Its job is to aid fatty acids into the powerhouse part of the cell or mitochondria. This will then lead to increased metabolic activity.

Vinpocetine: Vinpocetine will increase blood flow to the brain and help with protecting the neurons in the brain against injury.

Huperzine A: Also used to increase blood flow, it will act as a cholinesterase inhibitor, therefore it will increase the levels of acetylcholine.

Premier Pink Salt: Salt really gets a bad rap, yet we need it to survive. Salt is vital for a healthy nervous system. This unrefined, untreated sea salt is for everyday use. It has critical trace elements that are necessary for a healthy nervous system. This pink salt is *aleae* salt, from Hawaii; not to be confused with the pink Himalayan salt scraped from the walls of mines. Aways make sure that the salt that you are using is *not* filtered by metal screens as this can lead to metal toxicity. Always try to have unrefined salt that is sifted or filtered through wooden screens.

pH Salts: This supplement, available from Immunologic, has alkalizing mineral salts of calcium, magnesium, potassium, and sodium. It helps in supporting normal pH, which should be between 6.4 and 7.0. This should be used in conjunction with Ionic Mineral Drops.

Ionic Mineral Drops: Also from Immunologic, this is optimal for absorption and assimilation. It is a liquid concentrate of magnesium and potassium, calcium, boron, manganese, and gold. When used in concert with pH salts, it will stabilize the body's pH.

Methyl Folate Plus: This supplement from Neurobiologix contains two distinct forms of THF: methyltetrahydrofolate and folinic Acid. This helps those suffering from MTHFR gene problems. It also aids in recovery from neurological injury. www.neurobiologix.com.

Neuro-Immune Stabilizer: This exclusive formula from Neurobiologix is a topical solution that aids in immune function, mental focus and concentration, and effective hormonal regulation. This product is vital to support the methylation process associated with nervous system functions.

Vitamin D3: You may have heard about the properties of vitamin D for bones and teeth, but it is much more than that. Vitamin D is essential in the fight for maintaining a healthy immune system and cardiovascular support. In North America, most of us are deficient in this crucial vitamin. I recommend at least 5,000 IU to almost all of my patients.

Vitamin E: This vitamin is extremely important for cardiovascular health and for circulation. Vitamin E is available in many different forms and it is often misunderstood. This vitamin can search out and help to destroy free radicals. One of the best products that I have found is Deltanol from PR Labs. This product consists of four tocotrienols (alpha, beta, gamma, and delta). It is extremely helpful in decreasing inflammation.

Zinc: One of the most overlooked mineral in the body. It plays a vital role in antioxidation and the absorption and utilization of B vitamins. It is also vital for fetal and reproductive development.

When zinc is deficient or depleted, other metals take its place and cause an array of health conditions.

The following supplements are available from Premiere Research Labs, at www.prlabs.com:

Adaptogen-R3: This trademarked product promotes the adaptogeneic process, aiding the adrenal glands and supporting them on a daily basis.

Adrena Ven: This dietary supplement is a nutraceutical adrenal formula which gives comprehensive adrenal support.

Gallbladder-ND: This probiotic-derived formula is a botanical concentrate that delivers gallbladder support. It features the preferred forms of vitamin B6. Many people say that they can feel the difference the first time that they take it.

Green Tea: This is a strong antioxidant that helps with digestion and anti-aging. My preferred brand of choice is a liquid extract called Green Tea-ND.

Liver-ND: This is a wonderful probiotic-derived supplement that aids in detoxification and liver support.

Max B-ND: This supplement provides a great way to make sure that you are getting all of your essential B vitamins. Because the B vitamins are probiotic-cultured, they are rapidly delivered to the cells.

Nutritional Flakes Premier: This product is a superfood, rich in B-complex vitamins. It is a tasty source of high-quality, bioavailable protein.

Neuro-ND: This probiotic-cultured, live-source formula is vital for anti-aging, nerve, brain, and energy support.

Energy is often overlooked in our health and this product delivers it, while helping to fight off free radicals.

ThyroVen: This dietary supplement provides premier detoxification and thyroid support as well as comprehensive nourishment for healthy thyroid function.

The following biotics can be very helpful as well:

Dismuzyme: This free-radical scavenger uses *super oxide dismutase* (an enzyme that helps to quench free radicals). This product helps with inflammation and hepatic (liver) function and detoxification.

ADP: This Anti-Dysbiosis Product is based on oregano oil, a powerful anti-fungal and anti-microbial agent. It can break through biofilms of the cell to help with intestinal parasites such as SIBO and H. Pylori.

Bio Doph 7: This pre-biotic/pro-biotic will help replenish the gut with good microflora and decrease unfriendly organisms.

Cytozyme AD: Adrenal support that is derived from bovine (cow) neo-glandulars and is great for adrenal fatigue.

Gastrazyme: This is known for its gut-healing properties.

IPS Canada: Intestinal Permeability Support will help those suffering from leaky gut. It will also benefit those with Crohn's and gut dysfunction.

Disbiocide and FC Cidal: These are antimicrobials that help eliminate parasites.

Hcl Plus: For hypochlorhydria and systemic decrease in hydrochloric acid. It helps to support proper gastric function and proper food digestion.

These are some of the products that I use, but there are many others. Please make sure that if you are adding any supplements or nutraceuticals to your routine, that you are followed closely by your healthcare practitioner and follow their recommendations.

MANAGING YOUR DIET AND NUTRITION

You can support all the work of various therapies, medicines, and supplements by being aware of your food choices. Research foods that help and hurt autoimmune issues.

Try a prolonged period of adopting these guidelines to see whether you notice a difference.

The Autoimmune Protocol: What Can I Eat?

Fish, Poultry, Pork, Lamb, and Red Meat: You may eat as much beef, pork, lamb, wild-caught fish and poultry as you would like. If at all possible try to buy red meat that comes from organically raised, grass-fed animals.

Keep the fish to the smaller size to limit intake of mercury. Choices include shrimp, canned light tuna, salmon (canned, fresh, and frozen), pollock, haddock, oysters, sardines, tilapia, whitefish, and catfish.

Do not eat shark, swordfish, king mackerel, or tilefish because they contain high levels of mercury (US Food and Drug Administration, 2004).

Eat wild, not farmed fish, especially coldwater fish (wild salmon).

Stone Fruits and Berries: All fruits with a stone or pit. These include plums, cherries, peaches, nectarines, and apricots. Apples and pears may be consumed in limited quantities. Most berries are okay to eat (except those listed in the "do not eat" section of the guide).

Vegetables: All colors, raw, steamed, sautéed, juiced, or roasted. Choose organically grown whenever possible. If you can't get organic, then at least get your vegetables from local farmstands or farmers markets. Eat more vegetables than fruit.

Spices: Except those listed in the "do not eat" section of this guide, such as cayenne and paprika.

Oils: Olive oil and coconut oil can be used liberally. Cook with olive oil at low-medium heat, or use it cold. You may use coconut oil for higher temperature cooking. Unrefined coconut oil is stable up to medium-heat cooking and refined coconut oil is stable to medium-high heat cooking. You may also mix the two together to avoid smoking. Please avoid canola oil at all costs.

Saturated Animal Fats: Pork lard and beef tallow can be used in any dish.

Broth: Read the labels of store-bought broths for hidden ingredients. Try to use broth without salt and then add your own pink salt to taste. You can make your own chicken or bone broth.

Beverages: Drink plenty of water. You may add seltzer if you prefer. You may also add freshly squeezed lemon or lime to the water, but *absolutely no sugar*. Use only the juice; do not use the peel or rind.

Potentially Pro-Inflammatory

The foods listed below should be *avoided*:

- Nuts and any nut butters
- Eggs
- Coffee and black tea, both caffeinated and noncaffeinated
- Caffeine
- Alcohol
- Processed or canned foods
- Watermelon, mango, pineapple, raisins, canned fruits
- All sugars, including honey and molasses
- Mushrooms (they stimulate the immune system)

Do Not Eat Food List: What Should I Definitely Keep Off My Plate?

In order to maximize your healing, the following foods need to be *eliminated* from your diet:

All food that has gluten: The most common food allergies are caused by wheat and gluten-containing foods. Gluten is an amino acid that gives foods like bread their elastic properties and makes them chewy.

You will want to eliminate: wheat, rye, oats, and barley. These foods are found in bread, pasta, and other products containing refined flours. Wheat gluten is also added to many prepared foods as a binder, such as vegetarian and real sausage links, so please read labels carefully.

All grains: In addition to the foods above, cut out corn, rice, and other grains. Besides creating an inflammatory response, many of these ingredients in prepared foods come from sources that are genetically modified (see below for more information on GMOs).

All legumes, including beans, soy, and peanuts: Legumes contain estrogen mimics, which can be harmful to health. Beans, especially soybeans, but also favas and others, contain *phytoestrogens*. These mimic estrogen and can interfere with hormone function. Phytoestrogens evolved in plants as a defense mechanism, a way to disrupt the reproductive success of predators.

Legumes also contain *lectins*, a protien that binds to cell membranes. There is evidence that some lectins bind weakly to our cells' insulin receptors, like flipping a switch for cells to the *on* position for fat production and storage, which keeps you fat (Hedo et al., 1981).

All dairy (milk, cheese, yogurt, and yes, butter): Dairy products are a large source of allergies and many people have an underlying sensitivity to these. Dairy is one of the major causes of inflammation.

All refined sugar and anything containing it (chocolate, candy, condiments, and junk food): Refined sugar slows the process of detoxification in the body and has been shown to weaken the immune system. Sugars also cause the adrenal glands (stress organs) to work overtime, causing adrenal gland fatigue and altered blood sugar regulation.

Many processed or prepared foods, such as salad dressings and other condiments, gluten-free products, and expecially low-fat products have added sugar. Again, learn to read the ingredients of any packaged foods.

Nightshades (tomatoes, potatoes, peppers, eggplant, and tobacco): These are common allergy triggers and should be avoided because they can contribute to pain and inflammation. The nightshade or *Solanaceae* family also includes tomatillo, gooseberry, ground cherry, ashwaganda (winter cherry), and paprika. Many nightshades are in other prepared foods such as ketchup, pimentos, Tabasco and other hot sauces, salsas, chutneys, and relishes.

Corn: Much of the corn in the world has been genetically modified which in itself may cause an inflammatory response. But corn is also very high in fructose, high on the glycemic index, and therefore causes an excess release of insulin (a fat-storing hormone) and a pro-inflammatory response.

Soy: Also pro-inflammatory, as it increases levels of cytokines (IL-1,IL-6 and TNF alpha).

Cold cuts, bacon, hot dogs, canned meat, sausage, and shellfish: These meats should be avoided because they have been shown to increase inflammation. Most packaged, cured meats are full of nitrates and nitrites and should be avoided for the most part even if you don't have an autoimmune condition. Even the nitrate- and nitrite-free bacon, hot dogs, salami, pepperoni are still processed, so not the best choice for your protein.

Alcohol, caffeinated beverages (coffee, black tea, sodas), soymilk, and fruit drinks that are high in refined sugar: As we have seen throughout the book, the liver is an extremely important organ especially when in comes to detoxification and decreasing inflammation. Alcohol will affect this, as will beverages containing caffeine. They also cause increased adrenal production of cortisol resulting in poor blood sugar regulation and increased inflammation.

Unhealthy fats and oils, such as refined oils, margarine, shortening, and hydrogenated oils: The gallbladder and the liver are extremely hard hit by these products, so they should be avoided. I would avoid margarine altogether, no matter what condition you have. It is one molecule away from plastic and serves no benefit.

Distilled, white vinegar: Instead, use apple cider vinegar such as Bragg's Organic ACV.

All artificial sweeteners and/or flavorings: Many are excitotoxic, meaning that they induce nerve cell death. They also cause increased insulin release resulting in insulin resistant receptors on the cells thus being a cause of dysglycemia (altered glucose regulations) and diabetes.

Genetically Modified Organisms (GMOs)

Listed below are the products (and their derivatives) that are most likely to be genetically modified (GM).

Soybeans: (approximately 94 percent of U.S. crop in 2011) Genes taken from bacteria (*Agrobacterium* sp. strain CP4) are inserted into soybean DNA to make them more resistant to herbicides.

Corn: (approximately 88 percent of U.S. crop in 2011) Present in high fructose corn syrup, glucose, and some fructose, which is prevalent in a wide variety of foods in America. Corn that is sold directly to the consumer at roadside stands and farmers markets is most likely GMO. If you buy corn, only buy certified organic corn, popcorn, corn chips, and so on. In the United States and Canada, a food labeled "100 percent organic" is not allowed to include GMOs.

Rapeseed/Canola Oil: (approximately 90 percent of U.S. crop in 2011) Gene transferred into it to make crop more resistant to herbicide.

Sugar Beets: (approximately 90 percent of U.S. crop in 2010) Gene added to make crop more resistant to Monsanto's Roundup herbicide.

Cotton: (approximately 90 percent of U.S. crop in 2011) Cotton genes have been engineered to produce Bt toxin, a pesticide.

The seeds are pressed into cottonseed oil, which is a common ingredient in vegetable oil and margarine.

Dairy: Cows injected with GE hormone rBGH/rBST (growth hormones); as well as possibly fed GMO grains and hay.

Sugar: In 2012, the FDA approved GMO beet sugars to be sold on the market under the name: "SUGAR." So now, when we buy what's called "All Natural" Breyer's ice cream, we can't know for sure that we are eating regular or natural cane sugar. If you see "CANE SUGAR" there's a good chance it's not GMO.

Papayas: (most of Hawaiian crop; approximately 988 acres) In 1998, scientists developed a transgenic fruit called *Rainbow Papaya*. Now 77 percent of the crop grown in Hawaii is genetically modified.

Yellow Summer Squash and Zucchini: While the majority of squashes on the market are not GMO, approximately 25,000 acres of yellow summer squash and zucchini have been bioengineered.

Baked Goods: Often have one or more of the common GM ingredients in them. Why do we need corn or soy in our bread, snacks, or desserts? It's hard to find mixes to use as well. Some brands avoid GMOs (Bob's Red Mill, for instance). Find one you like and try to stick with it. Organic is one option; learning how to prepare brownies and other snack foods from scratch with your own organic oils is another.

Common Ingredients Derived from GMO Risk Crops: amino acids, aspartame, ascorbic acid, sodium ascorbate, vitamin C, citric acid, sodium citrate, ethanol, flavorings ("natural" and "artificial"), high-fructose corn syrup, hydrolyzed vegetable protein, lactic acid, maltodextrins, molasses, monosodium glutamate, sucrose, textured vegetable protein (TVP), xanthan gum, many vitamins, yeast products (Non GMO Project).

At a Glance: Foods to Include, Foods to Exclude

Here's a handy chart that will help you see at a glance which foods are the best to support your healing from autoimmune issues:

	Include	Exclude
Fruits	Stone fruits (avocado, peaches, plums, nectarines cherries, apricots) apples, pears and berries	All other fruits
Vegetables	All colors: raw, steamed, sautéed, juiced, or roasted	Corn, tomatoes, peppers, eggplant, mushrooms, white potatoes, GMOs
Starches	Rice, tapioca, quinoa, buckwheat, and millet are gluten-free, but limit their intake to begin with	Wheat, corn, barley, spelt, kamut, rye, oats
Legumes	No beans to begin with	NO SOY or soy products such as soy sauce, soy milk, tofu, tempe, nato, some vegetarian protein powders
Nuts and seeds	No nuts to begin with	Peanuts, peanut butter, cashews, cashew butter
Meat and fish	Fresh fish, chicken, turkey, wild game, pork, lamb, beef (grass-fed, organic is best)	Cold cuts, frankfurters, bacon, sausage, canned meats, eggs, shellfish
Dairy products	Milk substitutes (rice milk, almond milk, coconut milk, hemp milk)	Cream, yogurt, butter, ice cream, frozen yogurt, non-dairy creamer, margarine

Fats	Cold expressed olive oil, coconut oils, pork lard, beef tallow	Vegetable shortening, margarine, hydrogenated oils, mayonnaise, spreads, canola
Beverages	Filtered water, seltzer, mineral water	Soft drinks, alcohol, coffee, black tea, other caffeine-containing beverages, herbal teas
Spices	Ask your doctor — certain spices may trigger an immune reaction	Ketchup, mustard, pickle relish, chutney, soy sauce, barbecue sauce
Sweeteners (Not during the first 45–60 days of gut repair)	Brown rice syrup, fruit sweeteners, stevia, blackstrap molasses, xylitol Coconut palm sugar	White, brown, and refined sugars; honey, maple syrup, corn syrup, high fructose corn syrup, all artificial sweeteners

DYSGLYCEMIA AND REACTIVE HYPOGLYCEMIA

If you have *dysglycemia* or *reactive hypoglycemia* I suggest that you eat something every two to three hours. This helps to maintain stable blood sugar throughout the day and prevents cortisol (from your adrenal glands) and other stress hormones like epinephrine and norepinephrine from getting involved, which are released whenever your blood sugar begins to drop.

- Breakfast should be solely animal protein. If you are vegetarian or vegan, research good sources of high-protein, noninflammatory foods, such as protein powders derived from spirulina, hemp, or brown rice. At this stage, inflammatory nuts, legumes, grains, and gluten-filled foods like seitan or Textured Vegetable Protein (TVP) should be avoided. Sardines make the best first meal of the day due to their high omega-3 content and high protein yield. The ones packed in olive oil are the best and the only ones I know that are safe for us to eat. You can eat as much as you want of any animal protein, as long as it does not contain any of the forbidden foods or spices.

- One to two hours after your first meal, you may eat your carbohydrate and protein meal. I usually eat what I had for dinner the night before, or you may eat another breakfast with buckwheat or mixed vegetables.

- Two to three hours later could be your lunch, which is any of the approved vegetables along with animal-based protein.

- Two to three hours later, eat meat and vegetables again, any you like and as much as you like.

- Two to three hours later it's meat and vegetables, all you can eat.

- An hour or so before you go to bed eat a small meal consisting of mostly protein (at least 85 percent) and the rest vegetables.

A Few Tips

- If you need to have a snack, try stone fruits (fruits with pits) and fresh vegetables throughout the day if needed.

- Stay away from deep-fried foods.

- Bake or stir-fry your meals instead of frying or sautéing. This will help to keep the flavor and nutrients in the vegetables that you are using. Because the stir-fry uses fast, hot heat, it seals in many of the nutritive values of vegetables and proteins much more successfully than cooking for a prolonged period of time.

- Choose lots of colorful vegetables, especially lots of green, leafy ones.

- Staring your day off with a bowl of cereal is *not* the way to go. Eat protein for breakfast. Meats are a great option along with vegetables. If you want to stay vegetarian or vegan, investigate some of the protein powders available from plant sources that can either be blended with avocado or sprinkled over vegetables. Also consider adding spirulina or brewer's yeast to foods.

- Your meals are always to have at least some protein from animal sources if possible.

- Saturated fats are your friend; we are made of saturated fats. Try to remember that your brain, nerves, myelin, and sex hormones are made of cholesterol. Each cell in your body produces its own cholesterol, so don't believe that you are going to have high cholesterol because you eat meat.

- Drink plenty of water throughout the day. You may add fresh squeezed lemon to the water for added flavor, however, no juices or sugar is to be added.

- Go to www.ceceliasmarketplace.com/gluten-free-casein-free-soy-free-guide/ and purchase the Gluten-Casein-Soy-Free Grocery Shopping Guide.

- Always read the labels, even if you buy it often because you never know if they may change the ingredients.

- The easiest way to follow the initial portion of your program is to *eat only meat and vegetables*.

Special thanks to Dr. Josh Huffman and Dr. Walter Crooks in the creation of this chapter.

Case Study:

Multiple Autoimmune Diseases Case: Dr. Aubry Tager, DC (Burlington, Vermont)

Karen C. is a female in her forties who presented to my office with pain, numbness, and intermittent whiteness in her extremities (her hands and feet). This began back in 2009 and was made worse with exposure to the cold. She had a family history of autoimmunee disease in the form of ulcerative colitis. Her examination and history revealed a functional issue in the part of the brain (parietal lobe) that deals with sensory information. She also had some issues with her adrenal glands. She was acidic as well (not to be confused with pH of the blood which rarely changes).

We addressed the above issues with Max B ND, Vitamin D3 from PRL labs, GastroVen for her stomach, Nitric Balance from Apex Industries, and we decreased her acidic state with pH salts and ionic minerals from Immunologic. Being that she was diagnosed with Raynaud's disease, a form of autoimmunee disease, we also had to tackle the inflammation, which was done with CoCurcumin.

Her therapies included peripheral neuropathy rehab therapy via a rebuilder machine, cold laser to the extremities, neurofeedback via BrainPaint, and metronome therapy. This took place over the course of nine months and is still ongoing.

Here is what the patient had to say:

> I originally went to Dr. Tager to try to figure out why I was having Raynaud's attacks in my fingers. There was no way I could have known that the Raynaud's was only one of many symptoms that had manifested as a result of PTSD, including memory loss, concentration

issues, a large blind spot, decreased proprioception, and general malfunction in the right parietal region of my brain.

After a course of Dr. Tager's therapies, not only did the Raynaud's attacks substantially decrease, but my memory is much better, I am able to concentrate enough to where I am ready to go back to work, and my proprioception is markedly improved. The treatment has been nothing short of miraculous!

Conclusion

When I set out to write this book, the main purpose was for me to make sure that you are educated about autoimmune diseases. As somebody who suffers from an autoimmune disease, this is definitely something that hit home for me, and I wanted to make sure that you know there are different options available to you.

What are the important things to realize about chronic conditions—specifically, things like autoimmune conditions?

By the time you actually feel the symptoms, you already have the disease; in other words, it takes a while for the symptoms to develop. The problem has been going on for years, prior to seeing any kinds of signs or symptoms. This is what we call a *chronic condition*; it did not just happen recently as in the case of what we call an *acute condition*.

If it's chronic, it's something that's been going on for a long period of time. Because it is a chronic condition, it's going to take a lot of time, effort, and dedication on your part in order to see change. Unfortunately, there are no magic pills that are going to eliminate your autoimmune condition.

There are specific tests that we can do to find the causes. If we do this earlier on, then we're going to be able to make a bigger dent and bigger change in your life, rather than waiting for those symptoms to set in.

What the medical approach does is treat everybody the same way. They're looking at what types of symptoms you're presenting with when you come into an office.

When you visit your doctor's office, how do you feel, and what is your reason for being there?

Once they're able to piece together that symptomatology, the next process for them is to go to the PDR, or *Physicians' Desk Reference,* and come up with the appropriate medication to treat that. There are some medical doctors that will think outside the box, and are going to do things besides medication, but in general this is the approach that we see in North America. This type of approach doesn't really address or correct the underlying cause of the problem; you just end up chasing those symptoms around.

What we want to do is take more of a functional medicine or integrative medical approach. There's nothing more important than your immune system when it comes to outside invaders. To repel any kind of thing that's going to invade your body— whether it's a virus or any kind of bacteria—you need to have a functioning immune system. If your immune system is compromised, you leave yourself open to multiple threats. Once one does set in, there's the possibility of major complications developing. The first thing that we want to do is remove the triggers.

How are we going to do that?

Fix Your Gut

Eighty percent of the immune system is in the gut, and we want to make sure that we're eliminating any kind of problems where food particles may be leaking out through the gut, through these tight junctions that are there, through that mesh wiring that holds everything into the gut. If we keep that in check, that's going to allow the immune system to heal properly. We also want to make sure that we have the normal flora present in the gut. In your stomach, you have literally a trillion different bacteria. We want to make sure that we have more of the good ones, or the normal flora, as opposed to the bad ones.

Decrease Environmental Toxins

The next thing we want to do is make sure that we eliminate or decrease the amount of environmental toxins that are affecting our body. Last but not least, we want to look at any kind of metal toxicity. Metals are extremely toxic to our body, and if we can eliminate or decrease those, we're going to give ourselves a better environment in order to maximize our healing.

Regulate Your Blood Sugar Levels

You want to be able to handle your blood sugar level imbalances. If they're too high, you're going to make yourself susceptible to hyperglycemia, and that can lead to putting you into ketoacidosis, where your body becomes a lot more acidic.

That can lead to vision problems, it can lead to peripheral neuropathy, and eventually coma or possibly even death. We want to make sure that is kept in check. If you also have what's called hypoglycemia, where the blood sugar level is too low, then that also is going to be an issue, a little more quickly than hyperglycemia.

As the blood sugar level drops, you're going to lose your ability to focus. You might have some imbalance issues, have some dizziness, and then you could potentially pass out or also end up in a coma. If that's not taken care of, if there's not enough glucose being brought back into the body, that can also lead to incompatibility with life.

Build Your Immune System and Take Care of Your Brain

We are looking for specific things with regards to autoimmunity. We have to look at your thyroid and hormones. We have to look at the adrenal glands—your stress glands—and we have to address the liver. Last but not least we want to make sure that we are taking care of our brain.

Your brain is the computer for your body, and we want to make sure that everything is working properly with the brain. This is not a quick fix. You have to be ready, willing, and able to make a change.

Please remember what the point of this book is — it is not meant to debunk all of the medical information that you may have been given or taught. This information is meant to be informative and give you a call to action. Ask questions.

Ask your doctor:

"Why are you doing what you're doing?"

"What is the purpose?"

"What is the goal?"

"Are there any other options?"

If your current provider won't respond, or won't show you the way, then maybe they're not the right doctor for you. They might have different approaches to health, are too closed to outside ideas, or maybe they're just plain misinformed. Either way, if your current practitioner won't work with you or listen to your ideas, then I recommend you look for an alternative medical practitioner.

I can't stress this enough: We do not see quick fixes with autoimmune healing, and you must be ready, willing, and able to make the change. But when you are ready, we will be there for you.

Blood Values

TEST	Functional Range	Result: Norm, High, Lo	Function/Dysfunction
GLUCOSE	85–95 mg/dL	**Normal**	**The body's chief source of energy. It affects all organs, systems and tissues. It determines the acid/alkaline balance (pH).**
		High	Hyperglycemic tendency toward diabetes, lack of exercise, low thiamine, questionable diet.
		Low	Hypoglycemia, hypothyroidism, excessive insulin output, protein malnutrition.
URIC ACID	Male: 3.7–6.0 mg/dL Female: 3.2–5.5 mg/dL	**Normal**	**End product of protein utilization. Meat (esp. liver, kidneys), shellfish, and beans are high in uric acid**
		High	Gout, arteriosclerosis, rheumatoid arthritis.
		Low	Low B12, incomplete protein digestion, acidic pH, low in zinc and niacin.
BUN	13–18 mg/dL	**Normal**	**Reveals the degree of toxicity of protein to the kidneys.**
		High	Renal problems; dehydration; hypochlorydria (lack of stomach acid); high protein diet; stress; liver, thyroid, parathyroid imbalance; kidney obstruction (e.g., stones); low vitamin A, C, and/or E, potassium, abnormal blood loss.
		Low	Pregnancy, low protein or protein malnutrition, heavy smoking, tendency toward diabetes.

CREATININE	0.7–1.1 mg/dL	Normal	Relates to muscle activity and renal functioning.
		High	Dehydration; renal problems; enlarged prostate; indicates muscle breakdown to supply protein, high ingestion of meats, kidney distress.
		Low	Pregnancy, bone growth, stress to kidney (heavy coffee, tea, alcohol), too much vitamin C, compulsive exercise.
SODIUM	135–140 mmol/L	Normal	Essential to acid-base balance and intra- and extracellular fluid exchanges for normal body water distribution.
		High	Renal problems; need for water softener; high sodium diet; low water intake; relates to toxins, headaches, weak back muscles, low potassium levels, fluid imbalance, and lack of physical activity.
		Low	Low adrenal, low salt diet, lack of trace minerals, loss of fluids and loss of sodium in diarrhea or vomit.
POTASSIUM	4.0–4.5 mmol/L	Normal	Essential to heart and kidney function and the maintenance of pH of both blood and urine. Maintains regular heart rate and muscle force, thus helps to prevent heart and general muscle fatigue.

		High	Low adrenal; dehydration; low kidney function; overuse of potassium supplements; relates to congestive heart failure and renal failure, low vitamin E, insufficient exercise, and insufficient deep breathing.
		Low	Tissue destruction, high adrenal, renal problems, diabetes, tendency toward weak heart, alcohol-related folic acid deficiency, low fluid intake, low potassium intake, low vegetable and fruit intake.
CHLORIDE	100–106 mmol/L	Normal	**Indicates kidney, bladder, and bowel function. Essential for electrolyte balance and pH maintenance.**
		High	High adrenal, excess salt, renal dysfunction, high salt intake, severe dehydration, could relate to bowel dysfunction, insufficient green vegetables, liver malfunction, magnesium deficiency.
		Low	Low adrenal, low renal function, B12 deficiency, susceptible to infections, tendency toward colitis, bladder dysfunction.
CARBON DIOXIDE	25–30 mmol/L	Normal	**Bicarbonate is a vital component of controlling the pH of the body.**
		High	Alkalosis most commonly seen with lung disease or emphysema.
		Low	Acidosis can result in serious illness or kidney disease.

ANION GAP	7–12 mmol/L	Normal	Helps differentiate the causes of metabolic acidosis.
		High	Low thiamine, metabolic acidosis, kidneys.
		Low	Very rare.
CALCIUM	9.2–10.1 mg/dL9.7	Normal	About bone metabolism: the most important element in the body. Maintains cardiac regularity and is required for muscle relaxation and contraction; necessary for enzyme production; growth and development of teeth, bones, and resistance to infection.
		High	Excess vit. D use; excessive intake of milk, protein, antacids, or alcohol; bone disorders; possibility of calcium not being absorbed; lack of exercise or possible thyroid or parathyroid gland malfunction.
		Low	Pregnancy, osteoporosis, low thyroid or parathyroid gland malfunction, malnutrition, vitamin D deficiency.
PHOS-PHORUS	3.5–4.0 mg/dL	Normal	Critical constituent of all the body's tissues.
		High	Bone fracture, bone growth in children, renal dysfunction.
		Low	Hypochlorhydria (lack of stomach acid), low protein, low amino acid, vit. D deficiency.

MAGNESIUM	2.0–2.5 mg/dL	Normal	Critical to smooth muscle function, including heart, gastrointestinal tract and uterus; helps regulate acid-alkaline (base) balance in the body; aids in absorption and metabolism of minerals such as calcium, phosphorus, sodium, and potassium; also utilization of vitamin B complex, C, and E. Regulates body temperature.
		High	Low adrenal, renal dysfunction, low thyroid, infection.
		Low	Supplement use, malnutrition, alcoholism, and excessive use of diuretics.
TOTAL PROTEIN	6.9–7.4 G/dL	Normal	Screen for digestive problems, dehydration.
		High	Indicates a need for HCl, amino acids, and protein (indicates incomplete assimilation or non-use of protein); dehydration or loss of fluid.
		Low	Need HCl, amino acids, protein (incomplete protein digestion); poor nutrition; vitamin B, D, zinc deficiency.
ALBUMIN_	4.0–5.0 G/dL	Normal	Indicates blood vessel condition and fluid pressure.
		High	Dehydration, protein gram overload or absorption, hypothyroidism.
		Low	Starvation or malnutrition; edema; liver or kidney problems; vitamin C deficiency; hyperthyroidism; heavy aspirin use; liver, bile, decreased; immune function.

GLOBULIN	2.4–2.8 G/dL	Normal	Essential to the antibody-antigen response; needed to fight infections; important in blood clotting. Valuable in assessing degenerative and infectious processes.
		High	Hypochlorhydria (lack of stomach acid), allergy, a sign of arthritis.
		Low	Liver disease, inflammation, infection related, low protein digestion.
A/G RATIO	1.5–2.0 Units	Normal	Relates to the body's defense mechanism; associated with the liver.
		High	Not enough water before the test.
		Low	If below 1.1, check for pathogens.
TOTAL BILIRUBIN	0.2–1.2 mg/dL	Normal	End product of hemoglobin breakdown from red blood cells.
		High	Fat malabsorption and increased risk of cardiovascular disease, possible lymphatic problems, vitamin C deficiency, potential liver disease or jaundice, spleen dysfunction.
		Low	Iron deficiency, anemia, vitamin B12, C, and copper deficiency.
ALK. PHOS-PHATASE	70–90 U/L	Normal	Indicates how the liver is utilizing protein, fats, and pH balance (an enzyme found essentially in bone and liver).

		High	Bone growth (possible decalcification of bone), liver dysfunction, gastric inflammation, tendency toward arthritis, insufficient calcium/phosphorus, could relate to certain medications, bile duct obstruction, or alcohol related.
		Low	Protein malnutrition, vitamin C, folic acid and zinc deficiency, possible hypoglycemia.
LDH	140–180 U/L	Normal	**LDL is a catalyst for the conversion of pyruvic acid to lactic acid during cellular energy production.**
		High	Liver problems, cardiac stress, diabetic tendency, strenuous exercise, alcohol related, present in myocardial infarction and pulmonary conditions.
		Low	Reactive hypoglycemia, possible edema, fatigue.
AST (SGOT)	10–26 U/L	Normal	**Relates to liver enzyme activity, kidney and skeletal muscle.**
		High	Allergies, vitamin E deficiency, arthritic in nature, liver complications, heart or muscle problems.
		Low	Low B6 levels and magnesium deficiency.
ALT (SGPT)	10–26 U/L	Normal	**An enzyme associated with the liver, heart, and skeletal muscle.**
		High	Liver dysfunction, alcohol and drug related, vitamin A or C deficiency.
		Low	Low B6 levels.

GGTP	10–26 U/L	Normal	**An excellent indicator of liver damage or biliary obstruction of bile ducts outside the liver.**
		High	Alcoholism, bile obstruction, viral hepatitis.
		Low	Low B6 levels and copper, hypothyroid, low magnesium.
IRON SERUM	85–130 mcg/dL	Normal	**Critical to red blood cells ability to carry oxygen and remove carbon dioxide, helps to remove toxin residue from cells.**
		High	Hemochromatosis (excess absorption of iron), liver problems.
		Low	Iron deficiency, internal or external bleeding.
FERRITIN	Male: 33–236 Female: 10–122 Post-menopausal: 263	Normal	**The most sensitive test to detect iron deficiency. Main storage form of iron in the body.**
		High	Hemochromatosis (excess absorption of iron), acute malnourishment, infection, anoxia.
		Low	Iron-deficiency anemia.
TIBC	250–350 ul/dl	Normal	**Total iron-binding capacity. Measures the blood's capacity to bind iron.**
		High	Iron deficiency.
		Low	Hemochromatosis (excess absorption of iron).

HEMO-GLOBIN A1C	4.8–5.6	Normal	Measures blood glucose that has attached itself to protein (albumin). This test more accurately measures where glucose levels have been during the two to three weeks prior to the blood test.
	5.7–6.4	High	Increased risk for diabetes.
	>6.4	Very high	Diabetes.
CHOLES-TEROL	150–200 mg/dL	Normal	Fats that are made into hormones, enzymes and antibodies, lining of arterial walls. This is an effective measure of liver function, intestinal absorption, and cardiovascular disease.
		High	Diabetes, low thiamine, excessive dietary fats (hydrogenated oils), lack of vitamin A, C, D, E, stress, smoking, insufficient exercise.
		Low	Hyperthyroidism, protein malnutrition, alcoholism, excess carbs.
TRI-GLYCERIDES	75–100 mg/dL	Normal	Are major building blocks of very low density lipoproteins (VLDL) and play an important role in metabolism as energy sources and transporters of dietary fat.
		High	Dysinsulin, sugar and saturated fat eaters, stress related, increase risk of heart and small vessel diseases, poor exercise habits.

		Low	Nerves and stress related, protein malnutrition, excessive use of bran and niacin, low unsaturated fatty acids, hyperthyroidism.
HDL "GOOD" CHOLES-TEROL	>55 mg/dl– <80 mg/dl	Normal	**The good cholesterol, it carries cholesterol away from your arteries to your liver**
		High	Autoimmune condition, chronic liver disease.
		Low	Associated with angina pectoris and myocardial infarction, diabetes mellitus, lack of exercise, obesity, smoking, hypertension, and incomplete diet.
LDL CHOLES-TEROL	Less than 120 mg/dl	Normal	**The "bad" cholesterol, responsible for plaque build-up in the arteries.**
		High	As with Cholesterol/ Triglycerides.
CHOL/HDL RATIO	Less than 3.1	Normal	**It is the ratios between these substances that identify your risk of having heart problems. The lower the ratio, the safer you are.**
		High	Increased risk of having heart problems.
TSH	1.8–3.0 ulU/ml	Normal	**TSH stimulates the thyroid gland to secrete additional T4.**
		High	Hypothyroid symptoms.
		Low	Hyperthyroid symptoms (if less than 0.5).
FT$_3$	3.0–4.5 pg/ml	Normal	**This test measures the free or active T3 hormone (unbound) levels, which is the actual hormones that culminates in an increase in metabolism and energy.**

		High	Hyperthyroid symptoms.
		Low	Hypothyroid symptoms.
FT$_4$	1.0–1.5 ng/dl	Normal	**The measure of active T4 in the blood but must be converted to T3 to impact metabolism.**
		High	Hyperthyroid symptoms.
		Low	Hypothyroid symptoms.
T$_4$ TOTAL	6–12 mcg/dl	Normal	**Reflects the total output of the thyroid gland and actual T4 hormone released.**
		High	Hyperthyroid symptoms.
		Low	Hypothyroid symptoms.
T$_3$ TOTAL	60–180 ng/dl 0.6–1.81 ng/ml	Normal	**T3 is the most active thyroid hormone which is largely protein–bound but not necessarily available for metabolic activity.**
		High	Hyperthyroid symptoms.
		Low	Hypothyroid symptoms.
T$_3$ UPTAKE	28–38 mg/dL	Normal	**Indirect measurement of unsaturated binding sites on the thyroid binding proteins.**
		High	Hyperthyroid symptoms.
		Low	Hypothyroid symptoms.
REVERSE T$_3$	25-30 ng/dl	Normal	**Your body, especially the liver, can constantly be converting T4 to RT3 as a way to get rid of any unneeded T4.**
		High	Hyperthyroid symptoms.
		Low	Hypothyroid symptoms.
TPO AB	Above lab range 0–34	Normal	**Check in cases of autoimmune thyroid disorders.**

TGB AB	Above lab range 0–40	Normal	Check in cases of autoimmune thyroid disorders.
TH. BIND GLOB	18–27	Normal	This test measures the amount of proteins in the blood that transport thyroid hormones to the cells. Inherited thyroxine-binding globulin deficiency is a genetic condition that typically does not cause any health problems.
FTI FREE THYROXINE INDEX	1.2–4.9 mg/dL	Normal	The amount of unbound, physiologically active thyroxine (T4) in serum.
		High	Hyperthyroidism.
		Low	Hypothyroid, low levels of selenium.
WBC	5.0–8.0	Normal	Leukocytes, found in bone marrow. Protects body against infection and inflammation.
		High	Active stressed or compromised immune system.
		Low	Chronic stressed or compromised immune system.
RBC	Female: 3.9–4.4 Male: 4.2–4.9	Normal	Erythrocytes, relates to anemia. Carries oxygen to the cells and carbon dioxide back to the lungs.
		High	Polycythemia (a blood disorder in which your bone marrow makes too many red blood cells), altitude sickness, emphysema.
		Low	Iron deficiency, menses.

HEMO-GLOBIN	Female: 13.5–14.5 Male: 14–15	Normal	**Relates primarily to the liver and spleen. Indicates the amount of intracellular iron.**
		High	Altitude, hemochromatosis (an inherited condition, causes your body to absorb too much iron from the food you eat), pancreatitis, hyper-spleen reaction.
		Low	Menses or iron-deficiency anemias.
HEMA-TOCRIT	Female: 37–44 Male: 40–48	Normal	**Percentage of red blood cells to whole blood (plasma). Relates to abnormal state of hydration, also the spleen denoting the amount of blood cell breakdown.**
		High	Hemochromatosis, (an inherited condition, causes your body to absorb too much iron from the food you eat), spleen hyperactivity, mononucleosis, and dehydration.
		Low	Low vitamin B12 or Folic Acid; C, B-1, B-6, anemia; protein deficiency; improper diet; ulcerations; menses; or iron-deficiency anemias.
MCV	85–92 cu microns	Normal	**Average volume of many cells.**
		High	Anemia, B12 or Folic acid deficiency.
		Low	Iron deficiency, low B6.
MCH	27–32 cu microns	Normal	**A hemoglobin-RBC ratio, gives the weight of hemoglobin in an average red cell. Relates to iron, anemia.**

		High	Anemia B12 or Folic acid deficiency.
		Low	Anemia, Low B6, iron deficiency, need vit. C, internal bleeding.
MCHC	32–35%	Normal	**The volume of hemoglobin in an average red cell. Helps distinguish normally colored red cells from paler red cells.**
		High	Anemia, B12 or Folic acid deficiency.
		Low	Anemia, low B6, iron deficiency, need vit. C, internal bleeding.
RDW	Less than 13	Normal	**Indicator of red blood cell size.**
		High	B12/Folate anemia and iron anemia.
PLATELETS	50,000–450,000	Normal	**Cells in blood that form clots.**
		High	Polycethemia, free radical pathways, infection disorders.
		Low	Leukemia, immune dysfunction.
NEUTRO-PHILS	40–60%	Normal	**Amount of infection fighting capacity. The Good Guys.**
		High	Immune compromise, infections and poisonings, possible allergy, excessive amount of foreign protein due to undigested protein and muscle breakdown.
		Low	Low immune; free radical pathways; deficient vitamin A, B-6, B-12, folic acid, iron, and copper; toxin.

LYMPHO-CYTES	25–40%	Normal	**Aids in the destruction and handling of body toxins and by-products of protein metabolism. Relates to the healing process.**
		High	Stressed immune system, possible allergies, hepatitis, fever and infection.
		Low	Low immune, free radical pathways.
MONO-CYTES	Less than 7%	Normal	**Formed in the spleen and bone marrow, they can ingest and digest large bacteria. Related to normal tissue breakdown by the liver.**
		High	Inflammation, infection, parasites, BPH, possible viral infection, possible arthritis, stress, insufficient liquids.
EOSINO-PHILS	Less than 3%	Normal	**Responsible for the protection and preservation of life via the immunologic response. Relates to infections, inflammations, disease, and allergies.**
		High	Parasites, allergy, food allergies, intestinal infection, skin disease.
BASOPHILS	0–1%	Normal	**Involved in deep membrane allergies. Relates to the immune response, inflammation, and gastrointestinal tract.**
		High	Parasites, inflammation, possible allergies, hyperthyroidism, stress, blood complications E and C, blood clotting.

CRP C-REACTIVE PROTEIN	<1.0	Normal	Recent research suggests that patients with elevated basal levels of CRP are at an increased risk of diabetes hypertension and cardiovascular disease.
			Lower relative cardiovascular risk.
	1.0–3.0		Average relative cardiovascular risk.
	3.1–10.0		Higher relative cardiovascular risk.
VITAMIN B12	180–914 pg/mL SUFFICIENT	Normal	Vitamin B12 is required for proper red blood cell formation, neurological function, and DNA synthesis.
	145–179 pg/mL INSUFFICIENT	High	The symptoms of a vitamin B12 overdose are numbness and tingling in the hands and feet.
	<145 pg/mL DEFICIENT	Low	Anemia, fatigue, weakness, constipation, loss of appetite, weight loss, numbness and tingling in the hands and feet, difficulty maintaining balance, depression, confusion, dementia, poor memory, and soreness of the mouth or tongue.

VITAMIN D3 25-HYDROXY	30–100 ng/ml SUFFICIENT	Normal	Used to diagnose vitamin D insufficiency and monitor response to vitamin D therapy, controls the level of phosphate and calcium in blood, regulates bone health, invigorates the immune system, regulates neuromuscular functions, plays a vital role in cardiovascular functions, balances blood sugar level and insulin production, promotes normal cellular growth.
	10–30 ng/ml IN-SUFFICIENT		
	<10 ng/ml DEFICIENT	Low	Fatigue, general muscle pain and weakness, muscle cramps, joint pain, chronic pain, mood swings and depression, weight gain, high blood pressure, restless sleep, poor concentration, headaches, bladder problems, constipation or diarrhea, weak immune system, rickets in children.
VITAMIN D 1,25 DI-OH	10–75 pg/ml	Normal	The active form of vitamin D; order only for patients with hypercalcemia (too much calcium in the blood) or renal failure. Not used to diagnose vitamin D insufficiency.
		High	Abdominal symptoms: constipation; nausea; pain; poor appetite; Vomiting. Kidney symptoms: flank pain; frequent thirst; frequent urination.

HOMO-CYSTEINE:	Male: 6.3–15.0 µmol/L Female: 4.6–12.4 µmol/L	**Normal**	**Homocysteine is an amino acid in the blood.**
		High	Too much of it is related to a higher risk of coronary heart disease, stroke and vascular disease (fatty deposits in peripheral arteries).

**This chart is a guide for nutritional support information and to reinforce systemic and metabolic heath and is not intended as a diagnosis or treatment for any symptoms, conditions, or disease.

References

Ailioaie, C., et al. (1991). Beneficial effects of laser therapy in the early stages of rheumatoid arthritis onset. *Laser Therapy, 11* (2), 9–87.

Alfredo, P. P., et al. (2012). Clinical Rehabilitation. Efficacy of low level laser therapy associated with exercises in knee osteoarthritis: A randomized double-blind study. *Clinical Rehabilitation*, 26 (6), 523–533.

Alghadir, A., et al. (2013). Effect of low level laser therapy in patients with chronic knee osteoarthritis: A single blinded randomized clinical study. *Lasers Medical Science* (Aug. 3).

American Autoimmune and Related Diseases Association. (2016) aarda.org/autoimmune-information/autoimmune-statistics/

Bardot, J. B. (2013). Vitamin D3 plays significant role in slowing degenerative process in Multiple Sclerosis and CCSVI. *Natural News* (March 14). naturalnews.com/039480_vitamin_D3_multiple_sclerosis_CCSVI.html#ixzz4MpjkatfJ

Basirnia, A., et al. (1998). The effect of low power laser therapy on osteoarthritis of the knee. *La Radiologia Medica, 95* (4), 303-309.

Beth Israel Deaconess Medical Center and Harvard Medical School Teaching Hospital. What are the treatments for Crohn's disease? Accessed 8/12/16, www.bidmc.org/Centers-and-Departments/Departments/Digestive-Disease-Center/Inflammatory-Bowel-Disease-Program/Crohns-Disease/What-are-the-treatments-for-Crohns-disease.aspx

Beyer, Ed. (2012). How to get your life back from an autoimmune condition. Treating Fibromyalgia and Other Chronic Conditions Message Board (private message board). www.txfibro.com/

Bowden, J., & Sinatra, S. (2012). *The great cholesterol myth: Why lowering your cholesterol won't prevent heart disease – and the statin-free plan that will.* Beverly, MA: Fair-Winds Press.

Can MAP cause ulcerative colitis, as it does Crohn's? This Is Sussex. Accessed 8/12/16, communigate.co.uk/sussex/thechronicchronscampaignuk/page61

Coping with an arthritis flare. Arthritis Foundation. Accessed 8/12/16, arthritis.org

Dayan, C. M., & Daniels, G. H. (1996) Chronic Autoimmune Thyroiditis. *New England Journal of Medicine. 335* (2), 99-101. DOI: 10.1056/NEJM199607113350206

Edwards, C., J. (2008). Commensal Gut bacteria and the etiopathogenesis of rheumatoid arthritis. *Journal of Rheumatology.* August, 2008. jrheum.com/subscribers/08/08/1477.html

Fasano, A. (2001). Zonulin and its regulation of intestinal barrier function: The biological door to inflammation, autoimmunity and cancer. *Physiological Reviews, 91* (Jan. 2001), 151–175.

Greenstein, R. J. (2003). Is Crohn's disease caused by a mycobacterium? Comparisons with leprosy, tuberculosis and Johne's disease. *The Lancet, 3* (Aug.).

Grisanti, R. (2014). Fibromyalgia, who told you there wasn't a cure? Functional Diagnostic Medicine University. Accessed 8/12/16, functionalmedicineuniversity.com/public/986.cfm

Grisanti, R. (2016). Leaky Gut: Can this be destroying your health? Functional Medicine University. Accessed 8/12/16, functionalmedicineuniversity.com/public/Leaky-Gut.cfm

Grossman, A. B. (2012). Overview of adrenal function: Adrenal disorders. *Merck Manual*. Accessed 8/12/16, merckmanuals. com/professional/endocrine-and-metabolic-disorders/adrenal-disorders/overview-of-adrenal-function

Harvard Health Publications. health.harvard.edu/healthy-eating/glycemic_index_and_glycemic_load_for_100_foods

Health Library. Johns Hopkins Medicine. Accessed 8/12/16, www.hopkinsmedicine.org/healthlibrary

Hedo, J. A., Harrison, L. C., & Roth, J. (1981). Binding of insulin receptors to lectins: Evidence for common carbohydrate determinants on several membrane receptors. *Biochemistry, 20* (12), 3385–3393. DOI: 10.1021/bi00515a013

Hegedus, B., et al. (2009). The effect of low level laser in knee osteoarthritis: A double blind, randomized, placebo-controlled trial. *Photomedicine and Laser Surgery, 27* (4), 577–584.

Hershman, J. M. (2012). Overview of thyroid function: Thyroid disorders. In *Merck Manual*. Accessed 8/12/16, merckmanuals. com/professional/endocrine-and-metabolic-disorders/thyroid-disorders/overview-of-thyroid-function

Huan, C. et al. Diabetes mellitus and the risk of Alzheimer's disease: a nationwide population–based study.

Johnson, M. L. *Coffee enemas.* Accessed 10/9/16. youcanbeatthyroiddisorders.com/coffee-enemas/

Johnson, M. L. (2004). *What do you do when the medications don't work? A non-drug treatment of dizziness, migraine headache, fibromyalgia, and other chronic conditions.* 2nd edition. Appleton, WI: Jokamar-Jenake Publishing.

Jurgelewicz, M. Is there a relationship between lupus and vitamin D? (2012, May 15). Bucks County Center for Functional

Medicine. Accessed 8/12/16, thefunctionalmedicinecenter. com/2012/05/relationship-lupus-vitamin/

Kharrazian, D. (2010). *Why do I still have thyroid symptoms? When my lab tests are normal: A revolutionary breakthrough in understanding Hashimoto's disease.* Carlsbad, CA: Elephant Press.

Kleinewietfeld, M. (2013) Sodium chloride drives autoimmune disease by the induction of pathogenic T_H17 cells. *Nature* 496 (April 25). 518–522. DOI:10.1038/nature11868

Kuchinad, A., Schweinhardt, P., Seminowicz, Wood, P. B., Chizh, B. A., & Bushnell, M. C. (2007). Accelerated brain gray matter loss in fibromyalgia patients: Premature aging of the brain? McGill Center for Research on Pain. *The Journal of Neuroscience* (April 11).

Kwan, N. (2014). Oral contraceptives linked to increased risk of multiple sclerosis. *Fox News Health* (February 12). foxnews.com/ health/2014/02/28/oral-contraceptives-linked-to-increased-risk-multiple-sclerosis.html

Lievens, P., et al. (2002). The influence of low level infra red laser on the regeneration of cartilage tissue. *Lasers in Medical Science, 17* (4).

Mayo Clinic Staff. Fibromyalgia misconceptions: Interview with a Mayo Clinic expert. Mayo Clinic. Accessed 8/12/16, www.mayoclinic.org/diseases-conditions/fibromyalgia/in-depth/fibromyalgia/art-20048097

Mayo Clinic Staff. (2014). Hashimoto's disease causes. Mayo Clinic. Accessed 8/12/16, www.mayoclinic.org/diseases-conditions/hashimotos-disease/basics/causes/con-20030293

Nakazawa, D. J. (2009). *The autoimmune epidemic.* New York: Touchstone.

NCBI. Mycobacterium avium paratuberculosis and the etiology of Crohn's disease: a review of the controversy from the clinician's perspective. ncbi.nlm.nih.gov/pubmed/21037992

Non GMO Project. What is GMO? nongmoproject.org/learn-more/what-is-gmo/

Norwegian Health Technology Assessment Report. Norwegian Drug Agency.

Oz, M. (2009). Four treatments for fibromyalgia. *O Magazine* (Sept.).

Reese, D., et al. (2009). Neuromuscular electrical stimulation and dietary interventions to reduce oxidative stress in a secondary progressive multiple sclerosis patient leads to marked gains in function: A case report. *Cases Journal* (May). DOI: 10.4076/1757-1626-2-7601

Rosenfeld, G. & Bressier, B. (2011) Mycobacterium avium paratuberculosis and the etiology of Crohn's disease: a review of the controversy from the clinician's perspective. *Canadian Journal of Gastroenterology*. (Oct.) Accessed 10/9/16. ncbi.nlm.nih.gov/pubmed/21037992

Ruderman, E., & Tambar, S. (2012) Rheumatoid arthritis. American College of Rheumatology (Aug.). Accessed 8/12/16, rheumatology.org/I-Am-A/Patient-Caregiver/Diseases-Conditions/Rheumatoid-Arthritis

Shaw, G. (2009). Is fibromyalgia real? *Neurology Now, 5* (5), 29–32.

Scher, et al. (2013). Expansion of intestinal *Prevotella copri* correlates with enhanced susceptibility to arthritis. *eLife*. DOI: dx.doi.org/10.7554/eLife.01202.001

Stedman's Medical Dictionary, 26th ed. (1995). Baltimore, MD: Williams and Wilkens.

Stelian, J., et al. (1992). Improvement of pain and disability in elderly patients with degenerative osteoarthritis of the knee treated with low power light therapy. *Journal of the American Geriatric Society, 40* (1), 23–26.

Swenson, R. (2014). Chaper 8B. In *Review of clinical and functional neuroscience,* Dartmouth Online Education. Accessed 8/12/2016, www.dartmouth.edu/~rswenson/NeuroSci/index.html

Thomas, M. A., & Rosenblatt, D. (2005) Severe methylentetrahydrofolate reductase deficiency. In *MTHFR polymorphisms and disease.* Georgetown, TX: Landes Bioscience, 2005. 41–53.

Thyroid peroxidase antibody test: What is it? Mayo Clinic. Accessed 8/12/16, mayoclinic.org/thyroid-disease/expert-answers/faq-20058114

Trelles, M. A., et al. (1991). Positive outcomes for infrared diode laser in low reactive level laser therapy for knee osteoarthritis. *Laser Therapy, 3* (4), 149–153.

U.S. Food & Drug Administration. (2004). What you need to know about mercury in fish and shellfish. EPA-823-R-04-005. www.fda.gov/food/resourcesforyou/consumers/ucm110591.htm

Vitamin D supplements reduce pain in fibromyalgia sufferers (2014, Jan. 17). Elsevier. *Science Daily.* Accessed 8/12/16, sciencedaily.com/releases/2014/01/140117090504.htm

Vojdani, A. (2013). For gut's sake: Stop the autoimmune epidemic. Health Extravaganza Power Point (Anaheim). Accessed 8/12/16, media.scuhs.edu/extravaganza/speaker_ uploads/Dr._Vojdani_For_Guts_Sake_Stop_AI_Process.pdf

Weil, A. Fibromyalgia. Accessed 10/9/16, drweil.com/health-wellness/body-mind-spirit/autoimmune-disorders/fibromyalgia/

Weil, A. Rheumatoid arthritis. Accessed 8/12/16, drweil.com/drw/u/ART00663/rheumatoid-arthritis

Weill Cornell Newsroom. (2013) Toxin-Emitting Bacteria Being Evaluated as a Potential Multiple Sclerosis Trigger. weill.cornell.edu/news/pr/2013/10/toxin-emitting-bacteria-being-evaluated-as-a-potential-multiple-sclerosis-trigger.html

Weimer, L. H. (2003). Medication-induced neuropathies. *Current Neurology and Neuroscience Report* (Jan.).

Yacyshyn, B., Meddings, J., Sadowski, D., Bowen-Yacyshyn, M. B. (1994) Multiple sclerosis patients have peripheral blood CD45RO+ B cells and increased intestinal permeability. *Digestive Disease and Sciences (41)* 12, 2493–2498.

Zare, Y. Genetic basis of susceptibility to paratuberculosis infection in dairy cattle. University of Wisconsin–Madison, no. 3593497. Proquest Dissertations and Theses. Accessed 8/12/16, gradworks.umi.com/35/93/3593497.html

Zodkoy, S. (2014). *Misdiagnosed: The adrenal fatigue link.* Waitsfield, VT: Babypie Publishing.

About the Author

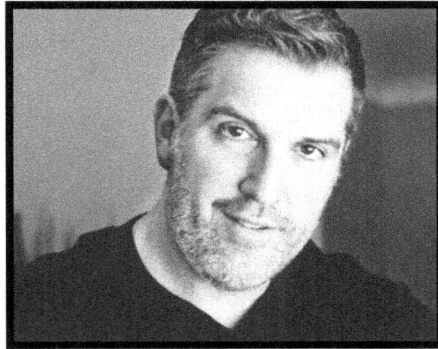

Dr. Aubry Tager is a native of Montreal, Quebec, Canada. He attended the University of Toronto for his undergraduate studies, and attained his Doctor of Chiropractic degree from Parker University (formerly Parker College of Chiropractic) in 1999. He completed the course work for the Diplomate of the American Board of Chiropractic Neurology, and is board eligible as a Functional Neurologist. "He holds the title of Doctor of Natural Medicine (DNM) through the Board of Natural Medicine Practitioners of North America and currently practices as a Naturopath through the association des naturopathes professionels du Quebec"

Dr. Tager strives to help his patients by staying current on the ongoing studies in the field of Neuro-Metabolic Care. He studied with Dr. Michael Johnson, Dr. Andy Barlow, Dr. Ted Carrick, Dr. Brandon Brok, and studied the works of Dr. Datis Karrazhian. He has achieved a post-doctoral Certificate from the American Functional Neurology Institute. He is a Diplomate through the American Association of Integrative Medicine and is Board Certified in Integrative Medicine. Dr. Tager is now an Executive Board member of the American Association of Integrative Medicine. He is currently completing a three-year Fellowship in functional neurology through IAFNR and National University of Health Sciences in Chicago, Illinois.

Dr. Tager offers frequent lectures and workshops on topics such as:

- Thyroid dysregulation
- Autoimmune disorders
- Peripheral neuropathy
- Fibromyalgia
- Concussions
- ADD/ADHD

He has been called as an expert witness in many depositions and court cases over the years as a result of his extensive knowledge.

In his spare time, he enjoys cycling, hockey, skiing, CrossFit training, and tennis. Dr. Tager is married to Doree Levine and has three children—Zach, Jordyn, and Cooper. He lives in Montréal, Québec. To learn more, visit www.neurologix.ca.

www.ingramcontent.com/pod-product-compliance
Lightning Source LLC
Chambersburg PA
CBHW072229270326
41930CB00010B/2052